The Cross Cultural Health Care Program

The Cross Cultural Health Care Program (CCHCP) was established in 1992 in Seattle, Washington with a grant from the W. K. Kellogg Foundation. From the beginning, the organization's goal has been to bridge the gap between underserved communities and services to improve health and well-being.

Now an independent 501(c)(3) nonprofit organization, CCHCP has become the nation's leader in training and resources to overcome language and cultural barriers to health and human services. Each year, CCHCP trains interpreters, providers, and trainers in health and human services locally and nationally. Widely acknowledged as the creator of the premier 40-hour medical interpreter training program in the nation, CCHCP is a pioneer in many other areas of cultural and linguistic competence. Published resources include a series of nationally respected medical glossaries, ethnic profiles of refugee and immigrant communities, training manuals, videos and research reports. CCHCP builds institutional cultural competence through training, assessment and community-centered research.

For further information please contact The Cross Cultural Health Care Program, 4700 42nd Ave SW, Suite 580, Seattle, WA 98116, phone 206.860.0329, **publications@xculture.org**, or http://www.xculture.org.

CCHCP Bilingual Medical Glossaries:

- Amharic
- Arabic
- Bengali
- Bosnian
- Burmese and Karen
- Cambodian Khmer
- Chinese (Mandarin)
- English
- French
- Haitian Creole
- Hindi
- Japanese
- Korean
- Lao
- Nepali
- Polish
- Portuguese
- Russian
- Somali
- Spanish
- Tigrigna
- Urdu
- Vietnamese

Acknowledgments

We would like to thank all CCHCP staff and volunteers for their contributions to this publication.

Translators

Primary translation by:
> U.S. Translation Company

Assistance from:
The translation was verified for cultural appropriateness by:
> Padam Rizal

Medical Reviewers

> Marty Babcock, RN, ARNP
> Elizabeth Plotkin, MD
> Thomas Wood, MD

Preface

Our catalog of bilingual medical glossaries was developed to support our Bridging the Gap medical interpreter training program. Bridging the Gap has aided the many dedicated individuals around the country who provide interpretation services to limited English-speaking patients in health care settings. In a field where misinterpretation and misunderstanding can be serious and even fatal, finding the "right words" to interpret or translate in medical terminology is a tremendous challenge. We hope this glossary helps in that valuable work. This Nepali glossary is our latest publication, designed to meet the needs of changing demographics.

Development of the glossary consisted of several important steps. First, interpreters, translators, health care providers, public health workers, and staff at CCHCP and CalOptima selected approximately 2,400 words commonly used during the patient-provider encounter. Second, these words were defined appropriately in English in ways they might be used during the patient-provider encounter. And third, these often complex biomedical terms or phrases were translated into Nepali. During this process we continued to learn more about language, how people use language, and about the process of translation.

An estimated 17 million people worldwide speak Nepali. In the United States, the recent influx of Nepali-speaking refugees from Bhutan has prompted a need to address language and health care access needs. Nearly all of these refugees speak Nepali as a first or second language. The United States began receiving this refugee group in 2008 and over 23,000 have settled here so far.

The terms and phrases included here range from very technical biomedical terms, such as *hysterectomy*, to less technical but equally challenging terms to translate, such as *shortness of breath*. Although every attempt was made to include the most common terms used during the patient-provider encounter, some may have been left out. This medical glossary is not definitive; it is only intended to provide a foundation in medical terminology.

Each medical term or phrase in the glossary is accompanied by an English definition. Each definition captures the meaning and use of a word or phrase in a biomedical context. These definitions were reviewed and edited by medical professionals. Be aware that many of these terms have additional meanings applicable outside of the medical field, and caution should be used with such terms.

For example, in this glossary the word *beat* is defined as "a single contraction of the heart." Outside of medicine, *beat* does not refer to the heart and could be defined as "to strike or hit repeatedly, or a single strike or blow." Selection of the correct terms to use in translations or interpretations is left to the interpreter, but keep in mind the definitions in this glossary focus on the way these terms are used in a biomedical context.

In every step of this process, the greatest challenge was translating terms out of context. Wolfgang Teubert, a German linguist, clearly explained this barrier in his article Translation and the Dictionary (Institut fur deutsche Sprache - The Tuscan Word Centre Workshop 19th - 21st June 1998);

> Looking at citations from the *Bank of English* (a dictionary), we again demonstrate the difficulty of selecting the proper translation equivalent for the words *sorrow* and *grief*. It seems that the problem with words like these is that they acquire their specific meaning only in connection with the context they occur in. The rules accounting for the selection of a particular word often differ from (English) to (Nepali). To choose the correct translation equivalent therefore means interpreting the (English) text in which the word in question occurs.

Throughout the glossary are symbols, word phrases, and annotations to help make the translation more transparent; that is, to help the users of this glossary understand how the translator came to choose words or phrases in the translation.

Nepali Medical Glossary User Guide

Basic Glossary Structure

Each entry in the glossary has several parts: In order, from left to right, they are 1) the English biomedical term or phrase, 2) the part-of-speech, 3) an indicator (m) if the word has multiple meanings in English, 4) the English definition, 5) the Nepali translation.

Several reference pages have been added at the end of the glossary, containing commonly used words in the categories of The Medical Team, Medical Specialists, Medical Procedures and Exams, Types of Pain, and Medical Equipment.

Excerpt from Medical Glossary

Term	Definition	Nepali
contusion (n)	a bruise, an injury of a part without a break in the skin	निलडाम

English Biomedical Term or Phrase

The first column of terms or phrases in the glossary represents our selection of nearly 2,400 biomedical terms commonly used during the patient-provider encounter. This word list is organized in alphabetical order and grouped by each word's first letter. Terms and phrases are presented in their proper lower-case form except for non-scientific or non-medical names of diseases, such as *Crohn's Disease.*

Several English terms or phrases are accompanied by an additional word or phrase in parentheses "( )". These additional words give the English word more context to how it is being used in this glossary. For example, the term *glasses* has the following entry:

> glasses (eye-) (n)   a pair of lenses mounted in a light frame, used to correct poor vision or to protect the eyes.

Including "(eye)" into the glossary entry helps specify *eye-glasses* instead of the plural version of glass, which is often defined as "a container used for drinking or consuming a liquid."

To provide additional clarity, some English terms are followed by another word or set of words. Often the provider will use this additional word interchangeably with the first term. For example, in the following entry for *allergy shots*:

> allergy shots, immunotherapy (n)   an injection to prevent an allergic reaction.

Allergy shots, in some instances, can be exchanged with *immunotherapy*. However, *immunotherapy* does not share the same definition as *allergy shots*. The interpreter or translator should be aware of the relationship between these words, but should use caution when substituting the second term for the first in translation or interpretation.

Part-of-Speech

Each term or phrase is assigned a part-of-speech that designates how it should be used in a sentence. The part-of-speech abbreviations are defined as follows:

n	noun
adj	adjective
v	verb
prep	prepositional phrase

Multiple Meanings (m)

As explained in the preface, you will find many words listed that have multiple meanings or usages associated with them. To denote this, several key word entries are marked with "(m)". Our definitions focus on their medical definitions.

English Definition

The English definition expresses the meaning of the term or phrase and how it should be used in a biomedical context. Each definition was designed to retain the specific and often technical meaning of a term or phrase while effectively expressing the meaning of the term or phrase so that it could be understood by the general reader. In order to achieve this, many of the definitions convey a broader meaning of the word then focus this definition, such as in the following definition of *poison*:

> poison (n)   a substance that causes injury, illness, or death, esp. by chemical means.

Other definitions are expressed through examples and synonyms. Words *italicized* in the definition are specific Latin classification names for organisms.

Abbreviations Used in the English Definition

e.g.	*exempli gratia*, for example
esp.	especially
i.e.	*id est*, that is
etc.	*et cetera*, and so forth

Nepali Translations

Naturally, in a glossary of this type, it is impossible to include all possible regional variations. Our aim has been to define medical terms so as to give the exact or closest equivalent for the English term, and to list as many synonyms as practical. We feel, with the exception of some highly technical terms, that the definitions are readily understandable anywhere in the Nepali-speaking world. Users of this glossary are encouraged to make annotations of regional translations as they become aware of them.

The glossary translates only the English terms or phrases located in the first column of words. It does not translate the definition of terms or phrases.

We hope this glossary will be helpful while interpreting or translating in the medical field. However, no translation is ever "perfect." We welcome comments about the translations, word list, and publication design. This will help us improve future translations of other language glossaries, and in the end, aid other interpreters and translators.

English-Nepali Medical Glossary – A

Term	Definition	Nepali
abdomen (n)	part of body between the chest and legs; the cavity of the human body containing the stomach, intestines, liver, gallbladder, pancreas, spleen, etc.; also called the belly	पेट
abdominal (adj)	of, or pertaining to the abdomen	पेटको
abnormal (adj)	not normal; contrary to the usual structure, position, behavior, or rule	असामान्य
abortion (n)	the premature expulsion of a fetus from the uterus, or removal of a fetus not capable of living, developing, or functioning successfully	गर्भपात
abrasion (n)	an area of body surface where skin is removed through some mechanical process	कोतारिएको
abrupt (adj)	sudden and unexpected	आकस्मिक
abscess (n)	a localized collection of pus in tissues, organs, or confined spaces	पिप
absorption (n)	the uptake of substances into or across tissues, e. g., skin and intestine	सोस्नु
abstinence (n)	a refraining from the use of food, stimulants, or sexual intercourse	संयम, परहेज
abuse (v) (m)	to use wrongly or improperly; to misuse a substance, e.g., alcohol, medicine, or drugs	दुरुपयोग, गालीगलौज, दुर्व्यवहार

English-Nepali Medical Glossary – A

Term	Definition	Nepali
access (n)	a patient's ability to obtain medical care. The ease of access is determined by several components, including the availability of medical services and their acceptability to the patients, the location of facilities, transportation, and hours of operation and cost.	पहुँच
accident (n)	an unexpected event	दुर्घटना
accommodation (n) (m)	adjustment, such as that of the eye for various distances	बसोबास, बासस्थान, *ब्रानिपनु*
accumulation (n)	the action or process of gathering together; state of being or having collected together	जम्माहुनु
ache (n)	a dull pain	दुख्नु
ache (v)	to suffer a dull pain	दुखाउनु
acid (n)	any substance capable of reacting with and dissolving certain metals to form salts, capable of reacting with bases to form salts, or which has a sour stinging taste	अम्ल
acidity (n)	the quality of being acid or sour; the trait of containing acid (hydrogen ions)	अम्लीयपना
acne (n)	an inflammatory disease of the hair roots or sebaceous glands, frequently used alone to designate common acne	डण्डीफोर, पिड्का
acquired immuno-deficiency syndrome (AIDS) (n)	disease due to infection with the human immunodeficiency virus (HIV)	यौनरोग, एक्वाएर्ड इम्युनो-डिफिसीयंसी सिन्ड्रोम (एड्स)
action plan (n)	a summary of what is intended to be accomplished	कार्य योजना

English-Nepali Medical Glossary – A

Term	Definition	Nepali
activate (v)	to set in motion; to create or organize	सक्रिय पार्नु
active (adj)	1. in motion, moving; 2. functioning or capable of functioning	सक्रिय
Activities of Daily Living (ADLs)	activities performed as part of a person's daily routine of self-care, such as bathing, dressing, toileting, transferring, and eating	दैनिक जीवनका क्रियाकलापहरु (ए.डी.एलस्.)
acuity (n)	clarity or clearness, especially of vision	स्पष्टता
acupuncture (n)	a traditional Chinese therapeutic technique whereby the body is punctured with fine needles	एक्युपंचर
acute (adj)	sharp, poignant; having a short and relatively severe course	तिब्र, सारो
adam's apple (n)	a large visible portion of the larynx located in front of the throat	रुद्रघन्टी
adaptation (n)	the adjustment of an organism to its environment	रुपान्तरण, सहजता
addiction (n)	the state of being dependent on a habit, especially strong dependence on a drug	खराब बानी, कुलत
adequate (adj)	satisfactory in quantity or quality; sufficient	पर्याप्त
adhesion (n)	the joining of two parts or surfaces, such as the joining of two opposing faces of a wound	टाँसीइनु
admit (v) (m)	to permit to enter; to have room for	स्विकार्नु
adolescent (n)	an individual between puberty and adulthood, mainly in the teenage years	किशोर, युवक

English-Nepali Medical Glossary – A

Term	Definition	Nepali
adrenal gland (n)	one of two glands located above each kidney that secretes hormones	एड्रेनल ग्रन्थी
adult (n)	a living organism that has attained full growth or maturity	वयस्क
Adult Day Center (ADC)	a center that provides a wide range of services for adults who need a protected environment and care from trained staff	वयस्क दिवा केन्द्र (ए.डी.सी.)
Adult Day Health Center (ADHC) (n)	ADHC provides an individualized treatment plan, nursing and personal care, restorative therapies (physical, occupational, and speech), maintenance therapy, psychological counseling, and nutritional counseling	वयस्क दिवा स्वास्थ्य केन्द्र (ए.डी.एच.सी.)
Adult Day Treatment Center (ADTC) (n)	a center that specializes in the treatment of people with psychological problems, including dementia, on a short-term basis	वयस्क दिवा उपचार केन्द्र (ए.डी.टि.सी.)
Adult Preventive Services (n)	services to protect adults from getting sick	वयस्क रोकथाम सेवा
adulthood (adj)	fully developed and mature.	वयस्कपना
advanced directive (n)	a legal document created by an individual stating his/her wishes; this document may be used to guide medical care during periods when the individual cannot make decisions for himself/herself	अग्रीम निर्देशन
advanced stage (n)	highly developed or far along in course	अति बिकसीत अवस्था
advanced-registered nurse practitioner (n)	senior ranking nurse capable of prescribing medicines	एडभान्स्ड-रजिस्टर्ड नर्स प्राक्टिसनर

English-Nepali Medical Glossary – A

Term	Definition	Nepali
adverse effect (n)	undesired result	प्रतिकुल असर
advice (n)	opinion about what could or should be done about a problem	सल्लाह, सुझाब
advocate (n)	a person who speaks on behalf of another in a public show of support	वकालत
aerobic (adj)	requiring oxygen	स्वास सम्बद्ध
aerobic exercise (n)	continuous and vigorous activity, such as running or cycling, that uses oxygen and builds endurance of the heart and lungs	स्वास सम्बद्ध व्यायाम
aerosol (n)	a solid or liquid drug carried in a fine mist for inhalation therapy	एरोसोल
affiliate (n)	an organization or person that directly or indirectly, through one or more intermediaries, controls, is controlled by, or is under the control of the contractor and provides services to or receives services from the contractor	सम्बद्ध, आबद्ध
affinity (n)	a special attraction for a specific element, organ, or structure	आकर्षण
afterbirth (n)	placenta and umbilical cord expelled from the uterus after childbirth	साल
agent (n) (m)	any power, principle, or substance capable of producing an effect, whether physical, chemical, or biological	प्रतिनिधि
aggravation (n)	an increase in seriousness or severity; an act or circumstance that intensifies, or makes worse	रोगले च्यापेको अवस्था
aggression (n)	hostile behavior	अतिक्रमण/आक्रोस

English-Nepali Medical Glossary – A

Term	Definition	Nepali
aggressive (adj)	the quality of being inclined to move or act in a violent or hostile manner	आक्रामक / *[handwritten]*
agitation (n)	a state of being upset; disturbance; commotion	व्याकुलता / *[handwritten]*
aid codes (n)	the two-digit number which indicates the aid category under which a person is eligible to receive Medi-Cal	सहायता संकेतलिपि
AIDS (n)	disease due to infection with the human immunodeficiency virus (HIV). AIDS is an acronym for Acquired Immuno-Deficiency Syndrome	एड्स
ailment (n)	a physical or mental disorder	बिमार / बिराम
air lift (n)	a system of transporting patients by air when surface routes are blocked	हवाई मार्ग बाट लानु
airway (n)	a passage in which air enters the body, e.g., trachea, bronchi, and lungs	श्वासनली
airway obstruction (n)	any object or substance that prevents breathing by blocking the passage of air into the lungs	श्वासनलीको रोकावट
albumin (n)	a type of protein	अल्बुमिन
alcohol (n)	a water soluble molecule; an intoxicating liquor	मदिरा
alcoholic beverage (n)	an intoxicating beverage; spirit	मदिरायुक्त पेय
Alcoholism (n)	a disorder characterized by excessive alcohol use that causes serious impairment in physical, social or occupational functioning	रक्सीको कुलत

English-Nepali Medical Glossary – A

Term	Definition	Nepali
alert (adj)	attentive and quick to think or act	सतर्क
alkaline (adj)	relating to or containing an aqueous solution that is bitter, slippery, and characteristically basic in chemical reactions	क्षारीय
allergen (n)	a substance that causes an allergy	एलर्जी गराउने बस्तु
allergic (adj)	causing allergy; having an allergy	एलर्जी हुनु
allergic reaction (n)	a physical response to an allergen	एलर्जीक प्रतिक्रिया
allergic rhinitis (n)	medical term for hay fever, a condition due to allergy that mimics a chronic cold	एलर्जीयुक्त रुघाखोकी
allergist (n)	a physician specializing in allergies	एलर्जी बिशेषज्ञ
allergy (n)	an extreme sensitivity to environmental factors or substances, such as pollens, dust, or foods, that causes a pathological response, such as a rash or difficulty in breathing	एलर्जी
allergy shots, immunotherapy (n)	an injection to prevent an allergic reaction	एलर्जीको खोप, इम्युनोथेरापी
alpha-fetoprotein test (n)	a test used to detect disease and some tumors in a fetus	अल्फा-फिटोप्रोटिन परिक्षण
alternate (v)	to change from one to another, sometimes back and forth	अगाडी-पछाडी पार्नु
alternative (n) (m)	something that is available in place of something else	बैकल्पिक
Alzheimer's Day Care Resource Centers (ADCRC) (n)	a center specializing in programs for persons with Alzheimer's disease or related dementia	अल्जाईमर्स डे केयर रिसोर्स सेन्टर्स (ए.डी.सी.आर.सी.)

English-Nepali Medical Glossary – A

Term	Definition	Nepali
Alzheimer's Disease (n)	a severe mental disorder marked by progressive decrease in intellectual capabilities	चेतना कमि हुने मानसिक रोग, अल्जाईमर्स रोग
ambulance (n)	a vehicle specially equipped to transport the sick or wounded	एम्बुलेन्स, बिरामि बोक्ने बाहन
ambulant (adj)	moving or walking about; having the ability to move	चल्न वा हिड्न सक्ने
ambulatory care (adj)	any type of health service that is provided on an outpatient basis	बहिरंग स्वास्थ सेवा
amenorrhea (n)	abnormal suppression or absence of menstruation	महिनाबारी नहुनु
American Academy of Ophthalmology (n)	an organization of opthalmologists (eye doctors) dedicated to providing comprehensive eye care	अमेरिकी नेत्र विज्ञान प्रतिष्ठान
American Cancer Society (n)	a nationwide community-based voluntary health organization dedicated to eliminating cancer as a major health problem by: preventing cancer, saving lives, and diminishing suffering from cancer, through research, education, advocacy, and service	अमेरिकन क्यान्सर सोसाइटि
amino acid (n)	an organic compound which is the foundation of any of various proteins, and is important for proper body function	एमिनो एसिड
amnesia (n)	lack or loss of memory; inability to remember past experiences	स्मरण शक्ती घट्ने रोग, बिर्सने बिमारी
amniocentesis (n)	the surgical withdrawal of a sample of fluid from the uterus of a pregnant woman	पाठेघरबाट तरल पदार्थको नमुना निकाल्नु
amniotic fluid (n)	the fluid surrounding a fetus	भ्रूणको वरीपरी हुने तरल पदार्थ

English-Nepali Medical Glossary – A

Term	Definition	Nepali
amphetamine (n)	a drug used to excite the central nervous system	एम्फेटामिन
ampoule (n)	a small glass or plastic container capable of being sealed to protect its contents from contamination	एम्पुल, इन्जेक्शनको सिसि
amputation (n)	the act or process of removing a body part, esp. an extremity including a finger, toe, hand, arm, foot, or leg	अंग बिच्छेदन
anaerobic (adj)	lacking molecular oxygen; growing, living, or occurring in the absence of molecular oxygen	अक्सिजन नहुँदाको अवस्था
analgesic (n)	a medication that reduces or eliminates pain	दुखाइ कम गर्ने औषधि
analysis (n)	an examination of a complex issue or substance by looking at the parts and their relations	बिश्लेषण, जटिल परिक्षण
anaphylaxis (n)	a high sensitivity to foreign substances	रोकथाम *अत्यन्त सम्बेदनसिल बाहिरि पदार्थ*
anatomical (adj)	pertaining to anatomy, or to the structure of the organism	शरीर रचना सम्बन्धि
anatomy (n)	any physical structure of the human body including organs, bone, muscle, and nerves	शरीर रचना विज्ञान
anemia (n)	a condition of an abnormally low number of red blood cells	रक्तअल्पता
anemic (adj)	suffering from anemia	रक्तअल्पतायुक्त अवस्था
anesthesia (n)	1. loss of feeling or sensation; 2. induced loss of pain, to permit surgery or other painful procedures	लट्याएको अवस्था
anesthesiologist (n)	a physician who studies and administers anesthetics	एनेस्थेसियोलोजिस्ट
anesthesiology (n)	the medical study and application of anesthetics	बेहोसीको औषधि बिज्ञान

English-Nepali Medical Glossary – A

Term	Definition	Nepali
anesthetic (adj)	a drug or agent that is used to abolish the sensation of pain	बेहोस बनाउने औषधि
anesthetist (n)	a person, usually a physician, trained to administer anesthetics	बेहोसीको औषधि दिने व्यक्ति
anesthetize (v)	to cause someone total or partial loss of sensation	बेहोसीको औषधि दिनु
aneurysm (n)	a sac formed in the wall of an artery, a vein, or the heart	धमनीविस्फार
angina (n)	a severe constricting pain in the chest	मुटुको दुखाई
angina pectoris (n)	a severe constricting pain in the chest, often extending from the chest to the left shoulder and down the arm, caused usually by heart disease	मुटुको दुखाई
angiogram (n)	an image of blood vessels created by injecting x-ray-visible fluid into the blood	एन्जिओग्राम, नसाहरुको तस्विर
angiography (n)	imaging of blood vessels following injection with a contrast material (visible by x-ray)	एन्जिओग्राफी, नसाहरुको तस्विर लिने काम
anguish (n)	an agonizing physical or mental pain; torment	पिडा, वेदना
ankle (n)	the joint, consisting of the bones and related structure, that connects the foot to the leg	गोलिगाँठो
anomaly (n)	marked deviation from the normal standard	असामान्य अवस्था
anorexia (n) (m)	lack or loss of the appetite for food	भोक नलाग्नु
antacid (n)	a substance that counteracts or neutralizes acidity, usually of the stomach	अम्लीयपना प्रतिरोधी औषधि
antagonist (n)	a drug that counteracts or neutralizes another drug	प्रतिरोधी औषधि

English-Nepali Medical Glossary – A

Term	Definition	Nepali
antecedent (n)	an event or thing existing or occurring previously	पूर्ववर्ती घटना
anterograde (n)	moving or extending forward; also called antegrade	अग्रगामी
antibiotic (n)	a drug used to treat bacterial infections	प्रतिजैविकी औषधि
anuresis (n)	the inability to urinate	पिसाबको रोकावट
anus (n)	the distal or terminal opening of the digestive system, through which feces are discharged	मलद्वार
anvil (n)	incus; small bone of the ear	कान भित्र हुने सानो हाड
anxiety (n)	a state of uneasiness and distress about something that is happening or may happen in the future, worry	बेचैनी, मानसीक रोग
anxiety disorder (n)	an illness with the following key symptoms: nervousness, apprehension, fear, worries	बेचैनी सम्बद्ध बिमारी
anxious (n)	worried and distressed about some uncertain event or matter; uneasy	बेचैन
aorta (n)	the largest artery in the human body; it carries blood away from the heart to the limbs	मुख्य धमनी
apathy (n)	lack of feeling or emotion; indifference	उदासिनता
aphasia (n)	defect or loss of the power of expression by speech, writing, or signs, or of comprehending spoken or written language, due to injury or disease of the brain	बोलि बन्द हुनु

English-Nepali Medical Glossary – A

Term	Definition	Nepali
aplastic anemia (n)	bone marrow disorder characterized by a reduction in the number of red blood cells, white blood cells, and platelets	एप्लास्टिक रक्तअल्पता
apnea (n)	absence of breathing	श्वासप्रश्वास रोकिनु
appeal (v)	a formal request by a patient or provider for reconsideration of a decision, such as a utilization review recommendation, a benefit payment or an administrative action, with the goal of finding a mutually acceptable solution	बिरामीको अनुरोध, रोगीको आग्रह
appendectomy (n)	the surgical removal of the appendix	एपेन्डिक्स काट्नु
appendicitis (n)	inflammation of the appendix	एपेन्डिक्स सुन्निनु
appendix (n)	a narrow worm-like appendage attached to the beginning of the large intestine	ठुलो आन्द्राको एक भाग
appetite (n)	a desire for food or drink	भोक
application (n) (m)	the act of bringing something into nearness or contact with another substance; the act of putting something to special use	लगाउनु, प्रयोग गर्नु
applicator (n)	an instrument used to apply a medication or substance	औषधी लगाउन प्रयोग गरिने औजार
appointment (n)	an arrangement to do something or meet someone at a particular time and place	नियुक्ति
aqueous (adj)	watery; prepared with water	जलयुक्त
aqueous humor (n)	a clear bodily fluid found in the eye	आँखामा हुने एक पारदर्शी तरल पदार्थ

English-Nepali Medical Glossary – A

Term	Definition	Nepali
arch (n)	a curved portion of the bottom of the foot	पैतालाको भित्रि भाग
arch support or insert (n)	an item used usually in a shoe to support the arch on the bottom of the foot	पैतालाको भित्रि भाग अड्याउनु
arm (n)	an upper limb of the human body connecting the hand and wrist to the shoulder	पाखुरा
armpit (n)	the hollow under the arm at the shoulder	काखी
arrhythmia (n)	any variation from the normal rhythm of the heart beat	धड्कनको असामान्यता
arterial (adj)	pertaining to an artery or to the arteries	धमनी सम्बन्धि
arteriography (n)	an x-ray of arteries after injection of material into the blood stream	धमनीको एक्सरे
arteriolosclerosis (n)	a chronic disease in which thickening and hardening of arterial walls makes blood circulation difficult	धमनी कडाहुने रोग
artery (n)	any of a branching system of tubes that carry blood away from the heart	धमनी
artery wall (n)	the inner surface that makes an artery	धमनीको भित्रि भाग
arthralgia (n)	pain in a joint	जोर्नीको दुखाई
arthritis (n)	inflammation of a joint or joints	जोर्नी सुन्नीनु
arthrogram (n)	an image of a joint after the injection of x-ray-visible fluid	जोर्नीको एक्सरे/तस्वीर
arthrosclerosis (n)	stiffness of the joints, especially in the aged	जोर्नीको कडापन
arthroscopy (n)	a procedure that allows direct examination of a joint using a small camera	जोर्नीको अवलोकन

English-Nepali Medical Glossary – A

Term	Definition	Nepali
articular (adj)	of, or pertaining to a joint	जोर्नीको
articular capsulitis (n)	inflammation of a joint capsule, such as the shoulder, knee, or elbow	जोर्नीको भित्रि भागको सुजन
articulation (n) (m)	1. the act or process of speaking; 2. the method or manner of joining; 3. a joint between two bones or between movable parts	बोल्ने प्रकृया, जोडाइ
artificial (adj)	not natural	कृत्रिम
artificial insemination (n)	the introduction of semen into the female reproductive organs without sexual contact	कृत्रिम गर्भाधान
ascending colon (n)	the first section of the large intestine	ठुलो आन्द्राको सुरुको भाग
asepsis (n)	absence of infection	संक्रमण रहित
aseptic (adj)	of, or pertaining to the state of being free of pathogenic organisms	संक्रमण रहित अवस्था
aspiration (n)	1. the act of inhaling; 2. withdrawal of fluid from the body	श्वास लिने कार्य
aspirator (n)	an instrument used to remove fluid from a cavity	शरीरबाट तरल निकाल्ने यन्त्र
assay (n)	1. a procedure to study a substance, esp. a drug; 2. a substance to be studied; 3. the result of such study	जाँच, परिक्षण
assist (v)	to give support or aid	सहायता गर्नु
association (n) (m)	1. the act of joining in a relationship; 2. the act of connecting or joining together; 3. the act of connecting in the mind or imagination	सम्बन्ध, जोडाई

English-Nepali Medical Glossary – A

Term	Definition	Nepali
asthma (n)	a chronic respiratory disease, often arising from allergies, and accompanied by labored breathing, chest constriction, and coughing	दम
asthmatic (adj)	pertaining to a person with or who suffers from asthma	दमरोगि
astigmatism (n)	faulty vision caused by defects in the lens of the eye	दृष्टिको कमजोरी
astringent (adj)	topical drug that causes contraction, often found in lotion	संकुचन गराउने औषधि
asymptomatic (adj)	showing or causing no symptoms	कुनै लक्षण नदेखिएको
at risk (adj)	refers to any service for which the provider agrees to accept responsibility to provide or arrange for the provision of medical services in exchange for the capitation payment, which, except for any contractually established "stop-loss" arrangement, shall be payment in full	जोखिमपूर्ण
ataxia (n)	loss or lack of muscular coordination	माम्शपेसीको संकुचन नहुनु
atelectasis (n)	lack of gas from part or the whole of the lungs	श्वासप्रश्वासमा अवरोध
atheroma (n)	1. fat deposits on the walls of medium and large arteries; 2. a sebaceous cyst	धमनीमा चिल्लोपदार्थ जम्मा हुनु
atherosclerosis (n)	*see arteriosclerosis*	धमनी कडाहुने रोग
athetosis (n)	a condition of endless slow involuntary movements	हात खुट्टाको कम्पन

English-Nepali Medical Glossary – A

Term	Definition	Nepali
athlete's foot, tinea pedis (n)	a contagious skin infection caused by fungi, usually affecting the feet and sometimes the hands, and causing itching, blistering, cracking, and scaling	छालाको रोग
atrium (n) (m)	1. a chamber; 2. chamber acting as an entrance to another structure or organ; 3. a specific section of the heart	मुटुको माथीको भाग
atrophy (n)	a wasting away; a reduction in size of a cell, tissue, organ, or part	आकार घट्नु
attack (v)	to use violent force	आक्रमण
attending physician (n)	a physician primarily in charge of a patient's care in the hospital and who oversees the medical practice of residents	कार्यवाहक चिकित्सक
Attention Deficit/Hyperactive Disorder (n)	biological disorder that causes the suffer to be easily distracted, impulsive, and restless, it occurs more frequently in boys than in girls	एकाग्रता नहुने समस्या
atypical (adj)	irregular; not conformable to the type	असामान्य
audiologist (n)	a person who studies hearing defects and their treatment	श्रवण रोग विज्ञ
auditory (adj)	pertaining to the sense of hearing	श्रवण
auditory nerve (n)	a nerve that sends signals to the brain, enabling someone to hear	श्रवण स्नायु
aural (adj)	pertaining to, or perceived by the ear	कानले थाह पाउने
auricle (n)	the external portion of the ear	कानको बाहिरि भाग
auricular (adj)	relating to the ear	कानको, कान सम्बन्धि

Term	Definition	Nepali
auscultation (n)	the act of listening for sounds within the body with a stethoscope, chiefly for determining the condition of the lungs, heart, and abdomen	स्टेथेस्कोप लगाएर सुन्ने कार्य
authority (n)	persons in command, specifically a governmental agency or corporation to administer a revenue-producing public enterprise	अधिकार, अधिकारी
autoimmune (adj)	related to or caused by antibodies	प्रतिरक्षा प्रणाली सम्बन्धि
autopsy (n)	the examination of a dead body to determine the cause of death	मृत्युपर्यन्त गरीने परिक्षण
autotransfusion (n)	a method of returning blood back into the body	स्वरक्ताधान
axilla (n)	armpit, underarm	काखी

English-Nepali Medical Glossary – B

Term	Definition	Nepali
baby bottle (n)	a bottle containing baby formula or another type of liquid to be consumed by a baby	दुधदानी
baby formula (n)	a liquid food containing required nutrients for a newborn baby	शिशु आहार
baby teeth (n)	the first set of teeth to grow in a baby	दुधेदाँत
back (n) (m)	the rear area of the human from the neck to the waist	ढाड
back of knee (n)	the region on the backside of the knee	घुँडाको पछाडिको भाग, घुडीखोप
back of neck, nape (n)	the rear area of the neck	घाँटीको पछाडिको भाग, घुच्चुक
backache (n)	a pain or discomfort in the region of the back or spine	ढाड दुख्नु
backbone (n)	the vertebrate spine or spinal column; the major support of the back in a human	मेरुदण्ड
background (n)	1. the circumstances and events surrounding or leading up to something; 2. a person's total experience, education, and knowledge	पृष्ठभूमि
bacteria (n)	*see bacterium*	जिबाणुहरु
bacterial infection (n)	a specific pathology caused by bacteria, causing injury to tissue	जिबाणुको सङ्क्रमण
bactericide (n)	an agent that destroys bacteria	जिबाणुनासक
bacteriological (adj)	pertaining to the study of bacteria	जिबाणु विज्ञान सम्बन्धि
bacteriostatic (adj)	inhibiting the growth or multiplication of bacteria	जिबाणुको बृद्धि रोक्ने औषधि

Term	Definition	Nepali
bacterium (n)	one of a group of very small organisms that can be free-living or parasites, and have a wide range of pathogenic properties; singular of bacteria	जिबाणु
bad breath (n)	an unpleasant smell originating from the mouth, caused by some foods and not cleaning the teeth	सास गन्हाउनु
bad taste (n)	an unpleasant flavor	नमिठो
balance (n)	1. the act of bringing or keeping equal; 2. satisfying proportion or harmony; 3. the ability to stand without falling; 4. the amount owed after a partial settlement, whatever is left over, remainder	सन्तुलन
bald (adj)	the condition of not having hair, esp. on the head	तालुखुइले
ball of foot (n)	the padded portion of the sole of the foot closest to the toes	बुढीऔंला नजिकको खुट्टाको भाग
bandage (n)	a strip of fabric or other material used as a protective covering for a wound or other injury	पट्टि
barium enema (n)	the use of barium to help obtain an x-ray image of the colon	बेरियमको एनिमा
barrier (n)	an obstruction	रोकावट
basal (adj)	pertaining to or situated near a base, esp. basal temperature used in family planning	आधार सम्बन्धी
base (n) (m)	in chemistry, the non-acid part of a salt; a substance that combines with acids to form salts	क्षार
bathtub (n)	a tub for bathing, esp. one permanently installed in a bathroom	स्नान टब

English-Nepali Medical Glossary – B

Term	Definition	Nepali
battered child (n)	a child that has experienced physical or mental abuse	दुर्व्यवहार गरिएको बच्चा
beat (n) (m)	a single contraction of the heart	धड्कन
bed of the nail (n)	the part of the finger or toe where a nail begins to grow	नङ निस्कने औँलाको भाग
bedbug (n)	a wingless, bloodsucking insect that has a flat, reddish body and a disagreeable odor and that often infests human dwellings	उडुस
bedpan (n)	a metal, glass, or plastic container for receiving human bodily waste	कोपरा
bedridden (n)	the condition of not being able to leave one's bed because of disease, injury, or illness	थलापर्नु
bedsore (n)	a skin ulcer caused by laying in bed for an extended period of time	ओछ्यानमा घोटिएर भएको घाउ
bedwetting (n)	involuntary discharge of urine while sleeping	बिस्तारामा पिसाव गर्नु
behavioral health care (n)	therapy aimed at modification of behavior	ब्यबहार सम्बन्धी स्वास्थ सेवा
belch (v)	to expel gas noisily from the stomach through the mouth	डकार्नु
belief (n)	the mental act, condition, or habit of placing trust or confidence in a person or thing	आस्था, विश्वास
belief system (n)	the organization and framework of a person or group's beliefs	विश्वास प्रणाली
Bell's Palsy (n)	a condition/disease characterized by a sudden loss of sensation and movement of the face, thought to be caused by a virus	अनुहारको पक्षघात
belly (n)	the stomach; the abdomen	पेट

English-Nepali Medical Glossary – B

Term	Definition	Nepali
belly button (n)	the navel; the scar on the abdomen left after the umbilical cord is removed	नाभी
belt (n)	a strap of leather or cloth worn around the waist and used to support clothing	पेटी
bend over (v)	to assume a position where the body is leaning over at the waist; to bow	निहुरिनु
beneficiary (n)	any person eligible to receive services agreed upon in a contract	अंशियार, हकदार
benefit package (n)	services offered by an insurer to a group of individuals under the terms of a contract	लाभ योजना
benign (adj)	not malignant; favorable for recovery	निको हुने किसिमको
Beri Beri (n)	a disease caused by a deficiency or lack of thiamine, an essential nutrient, and that produces numerous problems including neurological disorders	बेरीबेरी
beverage (n)	any liquid made for drinking	पेयपदार्थ
bewitched (n)	the condition of being placed under someone's power by or as if by magic; cast under a spell	बोक्सी लागेको, मोहनी लागेको
bifocal glasses (n)	glasses capable of assisting someone's vision at two different distances, usually for reading and for looking at distant objects	आधा भागमा पावर भएको आधामा नभएको चस्मा
big toe (n)	the largest toe on the foot	खुट्टाको बुढी औंला
bike helmet (n)	protective gear for the head worn as a hat	हेल्मेट
bilateral (adj)	having two sides, or pertaining to both sides	द्विपक्षीय

English-Nepali Medical Glossary – B

Term	Definition	Nepali
bile (n)	a bitter, alkaline, brownish-yellow or greenish-yellow liquid that is secreted by the liver, stored in the gall bladder, and discharged into the small intestines; it aids in digestion, chiefly by dissolving fats	पित्त
bile duct (n)	any of the passages in the liver that move bile from the liver and gallbladder to the intestines	पित्तनली
biliary (adj)	pertaining to the bile, to the bile ducts, or to the gallbladder	पित्तसम्बन्धी
bilirubin (n)	the orange or yellow substance in bile	पित्तमा हुने पहेंलो पदार्थ
bill (n)	an itemized list or statement of fees or charges	बीजक
biological (adj)	pertaining to biology	जैबिक
biological clock (n)	a biological mechanism responsible for the time-dependent aspects of a living organism	जैबिक घडी
biology (n)	the science of living organisms and life processes, including the study of structure, function, growth, origin, evolution, and distribution of living organisms	जीबबिज्ञान
biopsy (n)	the removal and examination, usually microscopic, of tissue from the living body, performed to establish precise diagnosis	बायोप्सी
birth (n)	the beginning of existence; fact of being born; the act of bearing young; the passage of a child from the uterus	जन्म

English-Nepali Medical Glossary – B

Term	Definition	Nepali
birth canal (n)	the canal through which the baby passes in birth	जननमार्ग
birth certificate (n)	an official document recording the facts of birth, including date, time, and place, and names of the newborn's parents	जन्म प्रमाणपत्र
birth control (pill) (n)	a pill for the prevention of unwanted pregnancy	गर्भनिरोध चक्की
birth date (n)	the day of one's birth, according to the calendar	जन्ममिति
birth defect (n)	any of numerous problems found with a baby at birth	जन्मदोष
birth mark (n)	a mole or blemish present on the body from birth	जन्मखत
bite (v)	to cut, grip, or tear with or as if with the teeth	टोक्नु
blackhead (n)	a plug of dried fatty matter capped with blackened dust and skin that clogs a pore of the skin	कालो डण्डीफोर
bladder (n)	a sac that stores fluid, such as urine or bile	थैली
bleed (v)	to lose blood	रक्तश्राव
bleeding nose (n)	to lose or emit blood from the nose	नाथ्री फुट्नु
blemish (n)	a coloring or defect of the skin caused usually by a bruise, pimple, or scar	छालाको दाग
blind (adj)	being without sight; sightless	अन्धो
blind spot (n)	a region of someone's visual field where the person cannot see	दृष्टिक्षेत्रको नदेखिने बिन्दु
blink (v)	to close and open the eyes	झिम्क्याउनु

English-Nepali Medical Glossary – B

Term	Definition	Nepali
blister (n)	a thin, rounded swelling of the skin, containing watery matter, caused by burning or irritation	फोका
bloated (adj)	a condition, feeling or sensation of being filled or swollen with water or air	फुलेको
block (n)	an obstruction or stoppage	अबरोध
blockage (n)	an obstruction or stoppage, esp. of a blood vessel or intestine	अबरोध
blood (n)	the fluid circulated by the heart through the vascular system that carries oxygen and nutrients throughout the body and transports waste materials to organs that will remove the waste	रगत
blood bank (n)	a place where whole blood is typed, processed, and stored for future use in transfusion	रगत जम्मा गर्ने ठाउँ
blood cell (n)	a red or white blood cell capable of transporting waste and oxygen or assisting in fighting a disease	रक्तकोष
blood clot (n)	a solid mass of blood	जमेको रगत
blood count (n)	the number of red and white blood cells in a specific volume of blood	रक्तकोषको गणना
blood culture (n)	a procedure of growing or developing blood cells outside of the body	शरीर बाहिर रक्तकोष विकास गर्ने काम
blood pressure (n)	the pressure of the blood within the arteries, primarily maintained by the heart	रक्तचाप
blood pressure cuff (n)	an instrument used to measure blood pressure	रक्तचाप नाप्ने यन्त्र
blood relative (n)	a person who is related by birth rather than by marriage	रगतको नाता भएको

English-Nepali Medical Glossary – B

Term	Definition	Nepali
blood serum (n)	the liquid part of blood	रगतको पानी युक्त भाग
blood sugar level (n)	the concentration of sugar (glucose) in the blood. It is usually measured in milligrams per deciliter (mg/dl)	रगतमा चिनीको मात्रा
blood sugar, glucose (n)	the amount of glucose and other sugars in the blood	रगतको ग्लुकोज
blood test (n)	an examination of a blood sample	रक्त परिक्षण
blood thinner (n)	a drug that helps prevent blood clots	रगत जम्न नदिने औषधि
blood transfusion (n)	the introduction of whole blood or blood component directly into the blood stream	रक्ताधान
blood type (n)	a system that categorizes blood according to specific chemical attributes	रक्तसमुह
blood vessel (n)	an elastic, tubular canal, such as an artery, vein, or capillary, through which blood circulates	रक्तनली
bloody stool (n)	feces that is red in color and contains red blood cells	दिशामा रगत आउनु
blow (v) (m)	to expel air from the mouth	फुक्नु
blurred vision (n)	vision that is hazy in outline or appearance; dim	धमिलो देख्नु
board certified (n)	refers to a physician who has passed an examination given by a medical specialty board and who has been certified as a specialist in that medical area	बोर्ड द्वारा प्रमाणित

English-Nepali Medical Glossary – B

Term	Definition	Nepali
board eligible (n)	refers to a physician who is eligible to take the specialty board examination by virtue of having graduated from an approved medical school, completed a specific type and length of training, and practiced for a specified amount of time	बोर्ड परीक्षाका लागि योग्य
Board of Directors (n)	a group of people who make policy decisions for an organization	निर्देशक मण्डल
body (n)	a group of organs and tissues working together to perform human functions; these functions include: the nervous system, circulatory system, respiratory system, skeletal and muscular system, digestive system, and the reproductive system	शरीर
body cell (n)	the basic unit or building block of all living matter that makes up organs that work together to perform major functions	शरीरको कोष
boil, carbuncle (n)	a painful, localized pus-filled swelling of the skin caused by infection	चाल्ने खटिरा, खटिरा
bone (n)	the dense, semi-rigid, porous, calcified connective tissue of the skeleton	हड्डी, हाड
bone fracture (n)	a partial or complete break in a bone	हड्डी भाँचिनु
bone marrow (n)	the soft material that fills bone cavities, consisting, in varying proportions, of fat cells, growing blood cells, supporting connective tissue and numerous blood vessels	हड्डीको मासी

Term	Definition	Nepali
bone marrow transplant (n)	the surgical procedure of transferring bone marrow from one human to another	मासीको प्रत्यारोपण
bone scan (n)	a procedure that uses radiation to diagnose bone diseases	हड्डीको तस्विर लिने काम
bone socket (n)	the hollow part of a joint that receives the end of a bone	हड्डीको खोपिल्टो
booster shot (n)	a supplementary dose of a vaccine injected to maintain immunity	अतिरिक्त खोप
bottle (n)	a container, usually glass, having a narrow neck and a mouth that can be plugged, corked, or capped	शिशी
bottle feeding (n)	a method of feeding a baby with liquid contained in a bottle, usually milk or baby formula	शिशीबाट खुवाउने काम
bowel (n)	an intestine, esp. of a human being	आन्द्रा
bowel incontinence (n)	a condition of being unable to control the evacuation of the bowels	दिसा नरोकीनु
bowel movement (n)	the passing of substances through the intestines	आन्द्राको चाल
brace (n) (m)	a device that holds or fastens two or more parts together or in place; clamp	काँटा लगाएर अड्याउनु
brain (n)	a portion of the central nervous system that is responsible for the interpretation of sensory impulses, the coordination and control of bodily activities, and the exercise of emotion and thought	गिदी, मस्तिष्क

English-Nepali Medical Glossary – B

Term	Definition	Nepali
brain damage (n)	injury to the brain that is caused by various conditions, such as head trauma, inadequate oxygen supply, infection, or intracranial hemorrhage, and that may be associated with a behavioral or functional abnormality	मस्तिष्कको चोट
break (v) (m)	to crack or split into two or more pieces with sudden or violent force, esp. a bone	भाँचिनु
break out (v)	to quickly develop (e.g., a skin rash, epidemic)	फैलनु
breast (n)	the human mammary gland	स्तन
breast cancer (n)	a tumor growth in a mammary gland	स्तन क्यान्सर
breast feed (v)	to feed (a baby) mother's milk from the breast; suckle	स्तनपान
breast mass (n)	a lump found on the breast, which may suggest cancer	स्तनको गाँठो
breast pump (n)	an instrument that assists the secretion and collection of milk from the breast	स्तन पम्प
breath (n)	the air inhaled and exhaled in respiration	श्वासप्रश्वास
breathe (v)	to take air in and out of the body	स्वास लिनु
breathing (n)	the act or process of respiration	श्वासप्रश्वास
breathing difficulty (n)	having a hard time moving air in and out of the body	श्वासप्रश्वासको कठिनाइ

English-Nepali Medical Glossary – B

Term	Definition	Nepali
breathing machine (n)	ventilator; an instrument that assists someone's respiration, ensuring that an adequate amount of oxygen reaches the lungs and that adequate carbon dioxide is removed	श्वासप्रश्वास सहज पार्ने यन्त्र
breech (n)	buttocks; lower rear portion of the body	नितम्ब
bridge of nose (n)	the hard upper part of the nose	नाकेडाँडी
broken (adj) (m)	of, or pertaining to a bone that has split or cracked into two or more pieces	भाँचीएको
bronchial (adj)	pertaining to one or more bronchi	सूक्ष्म स्वासनली सम्बन्धी
bronchiogenic carcinoma (n)	cancer originating in the bronchi	सूक्ष्म स्वासनलीको क्यान्सर
bronchitis (n)	inflammation of one or more bronchi	सूक्ष्म स्वासनलीको सङ्क्रमण
bronchopneumonia (n)	inflammation of the lungs, which usually begins in the terminal bronchioles	सूक्ष्म स्वासनलीको निमोनिया
bronchopulmonary (adj)	pertaining to the lungs and their air passages; both bronchial and pulmonary	फोक्सो तथा सूक्ष्म स्वासनली सम्बन्धी
bronchoscopy (n)	a slender tubular instrument with a small light on the end for inspection of the interior of the bronchi	सूक्ष्म स्वासनलीको अवलोकन
bronchospasm (n)	uncontrollable movement of the smooth muscle of the bronchi, as occurs in asthma	सूक्ष्म स्वासनलीको ऐंठन
bronchus (n)	either of the two air passages (pl. bronchi) beyond the windpipe that provide a way for air to enter the lungs	स्वासनलीको मुख्य दुइ हाँगा मध्ये एक

English-Nepali Medical Glossary – B

Term	Definition	Nepali
bruise (n)	an injury in which the skin is not broken; contusion	निलडाम
buccal (adj)	pertaining to or directed toward the cheek or mouth	मुखको
buckle up (v)	to fasten two strap or belt ends	पेटी लगाउनु
bulimia nervosa (n)	an insatiable appetite, often interrupted by periods of anorexia; bulimia is a psychological disorder that can be accompanied by self-induced vomiting	जति खाए पनि अतृप्त रहने
bullet (n)	a spherical or pointed projectile that is fired from a pistol, rifle, or gun	गोली
bullet wound (n)	the injury caused by a bullet	गोलीले बनाएको घाऊ
bunion (n)	a painful, inflamed swelling on the big toe	खुट्टाको बुढी औँलाको सुजन
burn (n)	an injury produced by fire, heat, or a heat-producing agent	पोलेको घाऊ
burn (v)	to damage or injure by fire, heat, or a heat-producing agent	पोल्नु
burning pain (n)	physical discomfort marked by intense heat	पोलाईले गर्दा दुख्नु
burning sensation (n)	feeling marked by intense heat	पोलेको अनुभूति हुनु
burp (v)	to belch, esp. after eating	डकार्नु
bursitis (n)	inflammation of a sac-like bodily cavity, esp. one located between the joints or at points of friction between two moving structures	जोर्नि भित्रको एक भागको सुजन
business office (n)	a location where a person engages in an occupation, work, or trade	ब्यबसायको कार्यालय

English-Nepali Medical Glossary – B

Term	Definition	Nepali
bust (n) (m)	a woman's chest; breasts	स्तन
buttock (n)	either of the two rounded, fleshy parts of the rump or backside of a human	नितम्ब
bypass (n) (m)	an alternative passage created surgically between two blood vessels, esp. to avoid an obstruction	उपमार्ग

English-Nepali Medical Glossary – C

Term	Definition	Nepali
caffeine (n)	a bitter substance found in coffee, tea, and soda, and used as a stimulant or diuretic	क्याफिन
calcium deficiency (n)	low levels of calcium in the blood preventing proper functioning of the body; see *deficiency*	क्याल्सियमको कमि
calcium(n)	a silvery, moderately hard metallic element essential to the proper functioning of the human body, found mostly in bone and teeth	क्याल्सियम
calculus (n)	a stone found in the body, esp. bladder, kidneys, urethra, and ureter; gallstone; kidney stone	शरीरमा हुने सानो पत्थरी
calf (n) (m)	the fleshy, muscular back part of the human leg between the knee and ankle	पिंडौला
callus (n)	a localized thickening and enlargement of the skin	छाला बाक्लिनु
calm down (v)	to become quiet; to lack or restrict movement; to become peaceful	शान्त हुनु
calorie (n)	any of several approximately equal units of heat, each measured as the quantity of heat required to raise the temperature of 1 gram of water 1 degree Celsius	ताप मापन एकाइ
cancer (n)	a disease in which cells grow and reproduce without regulation, these cells have a tendency to spread to other cells of the body	अर्बुदरोग, क्यन्सार
candidiasis (n)	a specific fungus infection	क्यान्डीडाको सङ्क्रमण
cane (n)	a stick used as an aid in walking	लौरी
canister (n)	a container used to hold fluid	गहिरो भाँडो

Term	Definition	Nepali
capillary (n)	the end of the smallest artery and the beginning of the smallest vein; the smallest blood vessel in the body	सुक्ष्म रक्तनली
capitation (n)	a contractual arrangement through which a health care provider or an HMO agrees to provide specified health care services to enrollees	स्वास्थ्य सेवा प्राप्त गरे बापत रकम तिर्ने एक पद्धति
capitation rate (n)	the amount paid per enrollee, per month, for services to be provided at risk.	स्वास्थ्य सेवा प्राप्त गरे बापत तिर्नु पर्ने रकमको दर
capsule (n)	1. a soluble container enclosing a dose of an oral medicine; 2. an envelope that encloses an organ or part in the human body	क्याप्सुल
capsulitis (n)	inflammation of a capsule	जोर्नीको क्याप्सुलको सुजन
car seat (n)	a device placed in an automobile, used to secure a child (under the age of six or under 45 pounds) when the automobile is in motion	कार सिट
carbohydrates (n)	a group of chemical compounds, including sugars and starches; major energy source of the body; also see *blood sugar*	कार्बोहाइड्रेट
carbon dioxide (n)	a colorless, odorless gas exhaled by humans as waste	कार्बनडाइअक्साइड
carbon monoxide (n)	a poisonous gas found in the exhaust of a car	कार्बनमोनोअक्साइड
carbuncle (n)	a specific inflammation or swelling of the skin that is accompanied by excretion of pus	पिपयुक्त खटिरा
carcinogen (n)	any substance that causes or increases the risk of developing cancer	क्यान्सर गराउने बस्तु

English-Nepali Medical Glossary – C

Term	Definition	Nepali
carcinogenic (adj)	of, or pertaining to any substance that causes or increases the risk of developing cancer	क्यान्सर गराउने बस्तु सँग सम्बन्धित
carcinoma (n)	a malignant new growth made up of cells tending to enter the surrounding tissues and spread throughout the body	क्यान्सर, ट्युमर
cardiac (adj)	pertaining to the heart	मुटु सम्बन्धी
cardiac arrest (n)	a sudden stop of effective pumping of the heart	मुटु धड्किन रोकिनु
cardiac catheterization (n)	a surgical procedure where a slender, flexible tube is inserted into the heart	मुटुभित्र नली घुसार्ने काम
cardiac scan (n)	a type of examination that studies heart function to assist in diagnosis	मुटुको अवलोकन
cardioangiography (n)	the process of creating an image of the heart and blood vessels around the heart by injecting an x-ray-visible liquid into the blood	कार्डियोएन्जियोग्राफि
cardiologist (n)	a person who studies diseases and functioning of the heart	मुटुरोग विज्ञ, मुटुरोग बिषेशज्ञ
cardiology (n)	the study of diseases and functioning of the heart	मुटुरोग विज्ञान
cardiopulmonary (adj)	pertaining to the heart and lungs	मुटु र फोक्सो सम्बन्धी
cardiopulmonary resuscitation (n)	a procedure employed after the heart stops beating in which cardiac massage, drugs, and mouth-to-mouth resuscitation are used to restore breathing	मुटु र फोक्सो सम्बन्धी समस्याबाट पुनर्जीवन
cardiorespiratory (n)	relating to the heart and lungs and their functions	मुटु, फोक्सो र श्वासप्रश्वास सम्बन्धी

43

Term	Definition	Nepali
cardiovascular disease (n)	disease affecting the heart or blood vessels; cardiovascular diseases include arteriosclerosis, coronary artery disease, heart valve disease, arrhythmia, heart failure, hypertension, orthostatic hypotension, shock, endocarditis, diseases of the aorta and its branches, disorders of the peripheral vascular system, and congenital heart disease	रक्तसञ्चार प्रणालीको रोग
cardiovascular system (n)	of, or pertaining to the heart and blood vessels / circulatory system	रक्तसञ्चार प्रणाली
care management (n)	a coordinated system of health-care services	स्वास्थ्यसेवा प्रबन्धन
caries (n)	the molecular decay or death of a bone	हड्डी खिईनु
carotid artery (n)	one of two arteries supplying blood to the neck and head	क्यारोटीड धमनी
carpal tunnel syndrome (n)	pain or loss of sensation in the hand and wrist caused by damage or overuse of the wrist	कार्पल टनेल सिन्ड्रोम
carrier (n)	a person who harbors a pathogen, and may transmit disease to others, without showing signs and symptoms of infection	रोग बाहक
cartilage (n)	a tough white connective tissue attached to the surfaces of bones	कुरकुरे हड्डी
case (n)	a situation, state of affairs, condition; a situation that requires examination	मामिला, स्थिति
case management (n)	method of managing health care services by which the medical, psycho-social, and other services are coordinated by one entity	मामिला प्रबन्धन
cashier (n)	the person in a business in charge of paying and receiving money	खजान्ची

English-Nepali Medical Glossary – C

Term	Definition	Nepali
cast (plaster) (n)	a rigid dressing, usually made of gauze and plaster of Paris, as for a broken bone	लगाइएको प्लास्टर
castration (n)	the removal of the testicles or ovaries	सुमर्ने काम, अण्डकोष वा डिम्बाशय निकाल्ने काम
casualty (n)	death of an individual; fatality	हताहत
cataract (n)	opacity in the lens of the eye, impairing vision or causing blindness	मोतिबिन्दु
catheter (n)	a tubular, flexible, surgical instrument for withdrawing fluids (or introducing fluids into) a cavity of the body	शरीरभित्र घुसाइने नली
catheterization (n)	the employment or passage of a catheter	शरीरभित्र नली घुसार्ने काम
catheterize (v)	to introduce a slender, flexible tube into a bodily channel, such as a vein	शरीरभित्र नली घुसार्नु
causal (adj)	pertaining to a cause; directed against a cause	आकस्मिक
caustic (adj)	capable of burning, corroding, dissolving, or otherwise eating away by chemical action	जलन गर्ने रसायन
cavity (dental) (n)	a pitted area in a tooth caused by caries	दाँतको प्वाल वा छिद्र
cecum (n)	the first part of the large intestine	ठुलो आन्द्राको पहिलो भाग
cell (n)	the smallest structural unit of an organism that is capable of independent functioning	कोष
cell membrane (n)	the structure enveloping a cell	कोषझिल्ली
Centers for Disease Control (CDC) (n)	a federal agency responsible for protecting the health and safety of people by developing and applying prevention and control of disease, injury, and disability	सेन्टरर्स फर डिजिज कन्ट्रोल (सी.डी.सी.)

English-Nepali Medical Glossary – C

Term	Definition	Nepali
cereal (n) (m)	a seed or grain high in starch and carbohydrates	अन्न, अनाज
cerebral (adj)	of, or pertaining to the cerebrum or the brain	मस्तिष्कको
cerebral palsy (n)	impaired muscular power and coordination due to brain damage, usually occurring at or before birth	पक्षघात
cerebrospinal (adj)	pertaining to the brain and spinal cord	मस्तिष्क तथा सुषुम्नाको
cerebrovascular (adj)	pertaining to the blood vessels of the cerebrum, or brain	मस्तिष्क तथा रक्तसञ्चारको
cerebrum (n)	the largest section of the brain	सेरिब्रोभास्कुलर
certificate (n)	an official document recording an event, achievement, or status	प्रमाणपत्र
Certificate of Coverage (COC) (n)	a description of the benefits included in a carrier's plan; the certificate of coverage is required by state laws and represents the coverage provided under the contract issued to the employer; the certificate is provided to the employee	सर्टिफिकेट अफ कभरेज (सी.ओ.सी.)
Certified Case Manager (CCM) (n)	a designation given to healthcare professionals what have formal training and "hands on" experience in the provision of case management services and processes	सर्टिफाइड केस म्यानेजर (सी.सी.एम.)
Certified Nurse Anesthetist (n)	a person licensed to assist an anesthesiologist	सर्टिफाइड नर्स एनेस्थेटिस्ट
Certified Nurse Midwife (n)	a person licensed to assist a pregnancy	सर्टिफाइड नर्स मिडवाइफ
Certified Nurse's Assistant (CNA) (n)	CNA assists the RN in the patient's care	सर्टिफाइड नर्सस् एसिस्टेन्ट (सी.एन.ए.)

English-Nepali Medical Glossary – C

Term	Definition	Nepali
cervical (adj)	pertaining to the neck, or to the neck of any organ or structure	पाठेघरको मुखको
cervical cancer (n)	cancer of the cervix, cancer of the entrance to the womb (uterus)	पाठेघरको मुखको क्यान्सार
cervix (n)	the constricted part of an organ, especially the opening into the uterus	पाठेघरको मुख
cesarean section (n)	a surgical incision through the abdominal wall and uterus, performed to extract an unborn baby	सेजारियन शल्यक्रिया
chamber (n)	a closed space, usually referring to a section of the heart	कोठा (मुटुको)
chancre (n)	a dull-red, painless ulcer that is the first evidence of syphilis	फोका
change your eating style (v)	alter or vary the way in which food is consumed	आफ्नो खाने तरिका बदल्नुहोस्
chart (n)	a sheet presenting information in the form of graphs or tables, esp. information about a particular patient	तालिका
check up (n)	a visit to a doctor's office for an interview and physical examination	जाँच, परिक्षण
cheek (n)	the fleshy part of either side of the face below the eye and between the nose and ear	गाला
cheekbone (n)	the bone just below the eye and above the fleshy part of the cheek	गालाको हड्डी
chemistry (n)	the scientific study of organic and inorganic elementary compounds and molecules	रसायनशास्त्र
chemotherapy (n)	the treatment of disease, esp. cancer, by means of chemicals	रसायनोपचार
chest (n)	the part of the body between the neck and the abdomen, enclosed by the ribs and the breastbone	छाति

English-Nepali Medical Glossary – C

Term	Definition	Nepali
chest hair (n)	hair located on the chest	छातीको रौं
chest pain (n)	an unpleasant sensation in the chest	छाति दुख्नु
chest x-ray (n)	a photograph of the chest, using x-rays, which produces an image of the lungs, ribs, and other aspects of the thorax	छातिको एक्सरे
chew (v)	to bite and mash food with the teeth	चपाउनु
chicken pox (n)	a very contagious disease, usually of young children, characterized by skin eruption and slight fever	ठेउला
Chief Medical Director (n)	a physician responsible for policy and procedures, and approval and denial of health--care services provided by a health plan or health network; he/she is also responsible for administrative matters of the health plan or health network related to health-care service delivery (in some health plans or health networks he/she may be called Medical Director)	प्रमुख चिकित्सा निर्देशक
child abuse (n)	the illegal act of physically or mentally injuring a child	बाल दुर्व्यवहार
Child Health and Disability Prevention (CHDP) (n)	a program which covers screening and diagnostic services to determine physical and mental defects in children under the age of 21 and to ascertain health care treatment and other measures to correct or ameliorate any defects and chronic conditions discovered	चाइल्ड हेल्थ एण्ड डिसएबिलीटि प्रिभेन्सन (सी.एच.डी.पी.)
childbirth (n)	the process of giving birth, or passing a child through the birth canal	बच्चा जन्माउने प्रक्रिया

English-Nepali Medical Glossary – C

Term	Definition	Nepali
chills (n)	a sensation of coldness, as with a fever	जाडो हुनु
chin (n)	the central forward portion of the lower jaw	चिउँडो
chiropractic (n)	a system of therapy in which disease is considered the result of incorrect alignment of bones causing poor function of the nerves; adjustments of the backbone and other structures is the preferred method of treatment	काइरोप्राक्टिक
chiropractor (n)	a person who applies chiropractic therapy	हाड तथा स्नायुको बैद्य
choke (v)	to prevent normal breathing, esp. by blocking the windpipe or by polluting the air	घाँटी अठ्याउनु, घाटिमा अडकीनु
cholecystectomy (n)	surgical removal of the gallbladder	शल्यक्रियाद्वारा पित्तथैली हटाउनु
cholera (n)	an acute, often fatal disease causing diarrhea, vomiting, cramps, and collapse	हैजा
cholesterol (n)	a pearly, fat-like substance that is a major cause of heart disease	कोलेस्टेरोल
chronic (adj)	persisting over a long period of time	जिर्ण, अती
chronic bronchitis (n)	a continuous inflammation of the bronchi	सुक्ष्म स्वासनलीको जिर्ण सुजन
chronic obstructive pulmonary disease (n)	a process that decreases the functioning of the lungs caused by numerous diseases	क्रोनिक अभ्ट्रस्टीक पल्मोनरी डिजिज
circulation (n)	the movement of blood through bodily vessels as a result of the heart's pumping action	रक्त सन्चालन
circulatory system (n)	the vessels, arteries, and veins, through which blood moves	रक्तसन्चार प्रणाली

English-Nepali Medical Glossary – C

Term	Definition	Nepali
circumcision (n)	the act of removing a section of the male or female external sexual organs	लिंगाग्रचर्म-उच्छेदन
cirrhosis (n)	a chronic disease of the liver marked by destruction and loss of liver cells leading to liver failure	सिरोसिस
classic (adj)	first class of rank; standard; well-known and typical	उत्कृष्ट, नमुना
classification (n)	the act or result of arranging or organizing according to class or category	वर्गीकरण
clavicle (n)	a bone that links the shoulder to the chest	काँधको हाड
clearance (n) (m)	the process of clearing; the rate at which a substance is removed from the blood	सफाई
client (n)	a person served by or utilizing the services of a social agency	ग्राहक
clinic (n)	an institution associated with a hospital or medical school that deals chiefly with outpatients; a medical establishment run by several specialists working in cooperation	क्लिनिक, स्वास्थ चौकी
clitoral (adj)	pertaining to the clitoris	भंगाकुरको
clitoris (n)	a small, erectile female sexual organ similar to the penis	भंगाकुर
clogged artery (n)	an obstructed or blocked artery	बन्द धमनी
clot (blood) (v)	to form into clots	रगत जम्नु
clot (n)	a thick mass or lump usually found in blood vessels	जमेको रगत
cloudy urine (n)	urine that is not clear	धमिलो पिसाब

English-Nepali Medical Glossary – C

Term	Definition	Nepali
clubbed fingers (n)	a condition where soft tissue in the fingers increases and fingernails curve in an abnormal way	हातको नङ कोप्रिने
coagulation (n)	the process of clot formation	रगत जम्नु
coccyx (n)	a small bone at the base of the spinal column	मेरुदण्डको तल्लो छेउमा हुने एक हड्डी
cold (illness) (n) (m)	common cold, a viral respiratory infection characterized by fever, chills, coughing, and sneezing	रुघाखोकी
cold sore (n)	a small ulcer or blister on the lips, usually accompanying a cold or fever	कोल्ड सोर
cold sweat (n)	sweat and chills happening at the same time, usually caused by fear, pain, or shock	गर्मी नहुँदा पनि पसिना आउनु
cold turkey (n)	a slang phrase used when people quit using an addictive substance all at once, without a period of gradual adjustment	लागूऔषधको बानी एक्कासी छोड्नु
colic (n)	acute pain in the abdomen, caused by spasm, obstruction, or widening of the intestine	शूल
colitis (n)	inflammation of the colon	ठुलोआन्द्राको सुजन
collapse (v)	to fall down; to cease to function; break down suddenly in strength or health	ढल्नु
collar bone (n)	the clavicle	काँधको हाड
colon (n)	the large intestine extending from the cecum to the rectum	ठुलो आन्द्रा
colonoscopy (n)	a procedure using a slender tubular instrument with a small light on the end for inspection of the colon	ठुलो आन्द्राको अवलोकन

Term	Definition	Nepali
color blindness (n)	an inability to see one or more colors	कुनै खास रंग देख्न नसक्ने अन्धोपन
colorectal cancer (n)	cancer of the colon and rectum	ठुलोआन्द्रा र मलाशयको क्यन्सार
colposcopy (n)	the examination of the vaginal and cervical tissues	योनीमार्ग र पाठेघरको मुखको तन्तुको अवलोकन
coma (n)	a deep, prolonged unconsciousness, usually the result of injury, disease, or poison	लामो अचेताबस्था
comatose (n)	pertaining to or affected with a coma	अचेत
combination (n)	a result or product of combining	संयोजन, मिश्रण
comfort (v)	to relieve or soothe pain during a difficult period	ढाढस दिनु
communicable disease (n)	a disease that is capable of being passed between people	सरुवा रोग
communication device (n)	a tool to help a person talk to another person	सञ्चार उपकरण
communication services (n)	services provided to help a person talk to another person	सञ्चार सेवाहरु
Community Alcohol & Drug Prevention (n)	public programs that offer education, support, and outreach resources to increase awareness of the dangers of alcohol and drug abuse	सामुदायिक मदिरा तथा लागूऔषध रोकथाम
Community Clinic (n)	a place in the neighborhood where people can come for routine health care services	सामुदायिक क्लिनिक
compatible (n)	capable of living or performing in pleasant combination with another or others; capable of forming a stable system	मिल्ने
compensation (n)	the act of making up for or offsetting; counterbalance	क्षतिपूर्ति

English-Nepali Medical Glossary – C

Term	Definition	Nepali
complain (v)	to express disappointment or dissatisfaction	उजुरी गर्नु
complaint (n)	an expression of disappointment or dissatisfaction	उजुरी
complementary (n)	forming or serving as a complement; completing	पुरक
complex (adj)	complicated, not simple	जटिल
complication (n)	a condition occurring during another disease and aggravating it	जटिलता
component (n)	a constituent element or part, as of a system	अंश
compress (n) (m)	a soft pad of gauze or other material applied to a part of the body to control bleeding or, moistened with water or medication, to reduce pain or infection	सेक्ने कार्य
computer axial tomography (n)	a diagnostic image of internal organs and soft tissue; also CAT scan	क्याट स्क्यान, सी.टि. स्क्यान
conceive (v) (m)	to become pregnant	गर्भधारण गर्नु
concentration (n) (m)	increase in strength by evaporation; the act of bringing a set of things closely together	एकाग्रता
conception (n) (m)	the first steps or beginning of pregnancy	गर्भावस्थाको सुरुवात
concomitant (n)	accompanying; accessory; joined with another	साथै आउने
concrete (n) (m)	solid, tangible	ठोस
concurrent review (n)	an assessment that determines medical necessity or appropriateness of services as they are rendered, such as an assessment of the need for continued inpatient care for hospitalized patients	समवर्ती समिक्षा

English-Nepali Medical Glossary – C

Term	Definition	Nepali
concussion (n)	a severe injury or shock, esp. to the brain	मगजको गम्भीर चोट
condition (n) (m)	1. the state of being or health of a person; 2. a specific ailment or disease	कुनै रोगको अवस्था
condom (n)	a sheath, usually made of thin rubber, designed to cover the penis during sexual intercourse to prevent pregnancy or the exchange of diseases	पुरुषले प्रयोग गर्ने परिवार नियोजनको साधन
conduction (n)	the transfer of sound waves, heat, nervous impulses, or electricity	संबाहन
confidential (adj)	done or communicated in secret; private	गोप्य
confusion (n)	disturbed orientation in regard to time, place, or person	अन्योल, भ्रम
congenital (adj)	of, or pertaining to a medical condition existing at, and usually before birth	जन्मजात
congenital heart disease (n)	a heart disease that existed at birth but is not hereditary	जन्मजात मुटुको रोग
congested, stuffed up (adj) (m)	having an accumulation of fluid in the lungs or nose	कुनै एक भागमा जम्मा हुनु, खाँदिनु
congestion (n) (m)	excessive or abnormal accumulation of fluid in a part	कुनै एक भागमा जम्मा भएको, खाँदिएको
congestive heart failure (n)	an enlarging and weakening of the heart caused by various heart diseases	कन्जेस्टिभ हार्ट फेलूअर
conjunctivitis (n)	inflammation of the mucous membrane that lines the inner surface of the eyelid and the exposed surface of the eyeball; pink eye	आँखा पाक्नु

English-Nepali Medical Glossary – C

Term	Definition	Nepali
conscious (n)	having an awareness of one's own existence, sensations, and thoughts, and of one's environment; capable of thought	सचेत, होसमा
consent (n)	to agree; to be of the same mind or opinion	सहमती
conservative (adj)	cautious	रुढीवादी
conserve (v)	to keep in a safe or sound state, preserve from change or destruction	रक्षा गर्नु
Consolidated Omnibus Budget Reconciliation Act (COBRA) (n)	A federal law that, among other things, requires employers to offer continued health insurance coverage to certain employees and their beneficiaries whose group health insurance coverage has been terminated	कन्सोलीडेटेड अम्नीबस बजेट रिकन्सिलेसन एक्ट (सी.ओ.बि.आर.ए)
constipated (adj)	experiencing difficult, incomplete, or infrequent release of feces	कब्जियत युक्त
constitutional (adj) (m)	affecting the whole body; not local	शारीरिक
consulting nurse (n)	a nurse that provides medical advice	परामर्शदाता नर्स
contact (n)	the coming together or touching of two objects or surfaces; a mutual touching of two bodies or persons	सम्पर्क
contact lens (n)	a thin corrective lens that fits on the eyeball	कन्ट्याक्ट लेन्स
contagious (adj)	passing by direct or indirect contact; carrying or capable of carrying disease	सरुवा रोग

Term	Definition	Nepali
contamination (n)	the act of polluting, soiling, or making something dirty; the act of giving something the ability to transfer a disease or cause an infection	प्रदूषण
contraception (n)	the prevention of conception or pregnancy	परिवार नियोजन
contraceptive (n)	an agent that diminishes the likelihood of or prevents one from becoming pregnant	परिवार नियोजनको साधन
contract (a disease) (v)	to acquire a disease	रोग लाग्नु
contracting providers (n)	a physician, nurse, technician, teacher, researcher, hospital, home health agency, nursing home, or any other individual or institution that an entity contracts with for medical services	करार प्रदाताहरु
contraction (n)	a shortening or reduction in size, esp. the shortening of muscle	संकुचन
contracture (n)	a drawing together, as of muscle or scar tissue, resulting in distortion or deformity	टेंडीएको, एकातिर तानिएको
contraindication (n)	any condition, especially any condition of disease, which renders some particular line of treatment improper or undesirable	निषेधित
contrast medium (n)	a substance that is introduced into or around a structure which allows a structure to become visible through x-ray	शरीरको अङ्ग स्पष्ट रुपमा देखाउन मद्दत गर्ने माध्यम
control (v)	1. to exercise restraint; 2. to have direct influence over; 3. to regulate, limit	नियन्त्रण

English-Nepali Medical Glossary – C

Term	Definition	Nepali
controlled drugs (n)	depressant and stimulant drugs that are frequently abused and must be prescribed for use by a physician	नियन्त्रित औषधिहरु
contusion (n)	a bruise, an injury of a part without a break in the skin	निलडाम
convalescence (n)	the stage of recovery following an attack of disease, a surgical operation, or an injury	स्वास्थ्यलाभ
conventional (adj)	traditional or customary	पारम्परिक
conversion (n) (m)	the development of repressed ideas or impulses in motor or sensory disorders such as paralysis	रूपांतरण
convulsion (n)	a violent involuntary contraction or a series of rapid movements	ऐंठन
coronary artery disease (n)	a pathology of the arteries that supply blood to the heart	मुटुको धमनीको रोग
coronary bypass surgery (n)	a surgical procedure that provides a new passage for a blocked coronary artery	मुटुको धमनीको शल्यक्रिया
coronary care unit (n)	a specially equipped area of a hospital providing intensive nursing and medical care for patients who have acute heart disease	मुटुरोग रेखदेख एकाइ
correction (n)	the act or process of removing errors or mistakes	सुधार्ने वा सच्याउने काम
correlation (n)	a causal, complementary, parallel, or reciprocal relationship, esp. a structural, functional, or qualitative correspondence between two comparable items	सहसम्बन्ध
correspond (n)	to be in agreement, harmony, or conformity; to be consistent or compatible	मेलखानु

English-Nepali Medical Glossary – C

Term	Definition	Nepali
corticosteroid (n)	any of the steroids made in the adrenal cortex	कोर्टीकोस्टेरोइड
cosmetic (adj) (m)	serving to beautify the body; decorative rather than functional	सौन्दर्य सम्बन्धी
cosmetic (n) (m)	a preparation, such as skin cream, designed to beautify the body by direct application	सौन्दर्य सामाग्री
cosmetic surgery (n)	a surgical procedure that corrects physical defects or non-functional aspects of the human anatomy	सौन्दर्यका लागि गरीने शल्यक्रिया
cotton (n)	thread or cloth manufactured from cotton fiber	कपासको धागो वा कपडा
cotton balls (n)	a small weave of cotton used to clean the skin	कपास
cough (v)	to expel air from the lungs suddenly and noisily	खोकी
cough drops (n)	a small, often medicated and sweetened lozenge or candy taken to ease coughing or soothe a sore throat	खोकीको गोली
cough syrup (n)	a medicated and sweetened liquid taken to ease coughing or soothe a sore throat	खोकीको झोल औषधि
counselor (n)	a person who gives counsel; adviser	परामर्शदाता
coverage (insurance) (n)	the extent of protection afforded by an insurance policy	बिमा
covered services (n)	health care services which are reasonable and necessary to protect life, to prevent significant illness or significant disability, or alleviate severe pain through the diagnosis or treatment of disease, illness, or injury, subject to utilization controls	जीवन रक्षाका लागि आवश्यक स्वास्थ्य सेवाहरु

English-Nepali Medical Glossary – C

Term	Definition	Nepali
CPT codes/coding system (n)	universally accepted billing codes [CPT = Current Procedural Terminology] utilized by healthcare providers for healthcare services and durable medical equipment (DME)	सी.पी.टि. कोड/ कोडीङ प्रणाली
cramp (n)	a sudden involuntary muscular contraction causing severe pain, often occurring in the leg or shoulder as the result of strain or chill	ऐंठन
cranium (n)	the portion of the skull enclosing the brain	खोपडी
crawl (v)	to move by using the hands and knees	घस्रनु
credentialing (n)	a process of review to approve a provider who applies to participate in a health plan; specific criteria and prerequisites are applied in determining initial and ongoing participation in the health plan	सेवा प्रदायकको योग्यताको समिक्षा
crippled (adj)	partly disabled or lame	अपाङ्गता
crisis (n) (m)	a sudden paroxysmal intensification of symptoms in the course of a disease	सङ्कट
criteria (n)	systematically developed, objective, and quantifiable statements used to assess the appropriateness of specific health care decisions, services, and outcomes	मापदण्डहरु
criterion (n)	a standard by which something may be judged	मापदण्ड
critical condition (n)	of, or pertaining, to a crisis	गम्भीर अवस्था

English-Nepali Medical Glossary – C

Term	Definition	Nepali
Crohn's Disease (n)	a chronic intestinal disease associated with inflammation of the small intestines	सानो आन्द्राको सङ्क्रमण हुने रोग
cross-eyed (adj)	having eyes that look in toward the nose	डेरो आँखा
crotch (n)	the region of the angle formed by the junction of the legs	दूई खुट्टा जोडिएको ठाउँको काप
croup (n)	a pathological condition affecting the larynx in children, characterized by respiratory difficulty and a harsh cough	केटाकेटीलाई लाग्ने एक प्रकारको श्वासप्रश्वासको रोग
crown (dental) (n) (m)	an artificial substitute for the part of the tooth above the gum line	गिजाभन्दा माथिको दाँतको भाग
crutch (n)	a device used to aid a paralyzed, weak, or injured person, usually a long stick or staff placed under the arm for support	बैशाखी
cryosurgery (n)	the selective exposure of tissues to extreme cold to bring about cell destruction	अत्याधिक चिसोले तन्तुहरू नष्ट गर्नु
cryotherapy (n)	application of liquid nitrogen; the use of low temperatures in medical therapy	अत्याधिक चिसोले उपचार गर्नु
crystallization (n)	the formation of crystals	त्रिआयामिक अणु वा परमाणु बनाउनु
crystals (n)	a three-dimensional atomic, ionic, or molecular structure consisting of periodically repeated, identically constituted, congruent unit cells	त्रिआयामिक अणु वा परमाणु
culture (n) (m)	the growing of microorganisms in a small dish	प्रयोगशालामा सुक्ष्म जिबाणु उमार्नु
cumulative (adj)	increasing or growing by accumulation or successive additions	संचित, जम्मा

English-Nepali Medical Glossary – C

Term	Definition	Nepali
curative (n)	an agent that helps overcome a disease and promote recovery	उपचारात्मक
cure (n)	a method or course of medical treatment used to restore health; an agent, such as a drug, that restores health; remedy	उपचार
curettage (n)	the removal of growths or other material from the wall of a cavity or other surface	खुर्केर हटाउनु
curve (n)	a line that deviates from straightness in a smooth, continuous fashion	वक्र, घुमेको
Customer Service Department (n)	a group of people organized and working together under a leader, and responsible for providing services (information, referral, and problem resolution) to patients, doctors, community, advocates, and others as needed	ग्राहक सेवा बिभाग
cut (n)	the result of cutting; an incision; the act of incising, severing, or separating	काटेको
cut (v)	to penetrate with a sharp edge; strike a narrow opening in	काट्नु
cutaneous (adj)	pertaining to the skin; dermal; dermic	छालाको
cuticle (n)	the strip of hardened skin at the base of a fingernail or toenail	नङको तल हुने कडा छाला
cyanosis (n)	a bluish discoloration of the skin, resulting from inadequate oxygenation of the blood	निलोपना
cycle (n)	a time interval in which a characteristic, esp. a regularly repeated, event or sequence of events occurs	चक्र
cyclic (adj)	of, or pertaining to, or occurring in a cycle or cycles	चक्रीय

Term	Definition	Nepali
cycloplegia (n)	inability to focus because of paralysis of the ciliary muscles of the eye	राम्रो सँग नदेख्नु
cyst (n)	any closed cavity or sac	थैली
cystic fibrosis (n)	a congenital disease causing chronic obstructive pulmonary disease and problems with the pancreas	सिस्टिक फाईब्रोसिस्
cystitis (n)	inflammation of the urinary bladder	पिसाबथैलीको सुजन
cystoscopy (n)	direct visual examination of the urinary tract with a tubular instrument fitted with a light	पिसाबथैलीको अबलोकन

English-Nepali Medical Glossary – D

Term	Definition	Nepali
damage (n)	impairment of the usefulness or value of person or property; harm	क्षति, हानि
dandruff (n)	white scaly skin that develops on and is shed from the head	चायाँ
danger (n)	a situation or condition that is harmful and may cause injury	खतरा
dangerous (adj)	of, or pertaining to a situation or condition that is harmful and may cause injury	खतरनाक
dazed (adj)	in a confused mental state	अन्यौलग्रस्त
deaf (adj)	partially or completely incapable of hearing	बहिरो
deafness (n)	the state of being partially or completely incapable of hearing	बहिरोपना
death (n)	the act of dying; state of being dead	मृत्यु
death certificate (n)	an official document recording the time, date, and location of a person's death	मृत्यु प्रमाणपत्र
decay (v)	to decompose, rot	कुहिनु
decompensation (n)	any process or mechanism to adjust or compensate; process of getting worse	परिपूर्ति गर्ने एक प्रक्रिया
decompression (n)	the act or process of relieving pressure; a surgical procedure used to relieve pressure on an organ or part	दबाब कम गर्ने एक प्रक्रिया
decongestant (n)	a medication or treatment that breaks up congestion, as of the sinuses	खुलाउने (जस्तै बन्द नाक) औषधि
deep (adj)	extending far downward below a surface; extending far inward from an outer surface	गहिरो

English-Nepali Medical Glossary – D

Term	Definition	Nepali
deep breathing (v)	the act or process of slowly allowing air to come through the nostrils and fill up the lower abdomen and then having the air escape through pursed lips	गहिरो स्वास लिनु
defecate (v)	to excrete or release feces from the bowels	दिशा गर्नु
deferred (v)	to delay an action or proceeding	स्थगित गरिएको
defibrillation (n)	the act of correcting an irregular heart beat by applying electric shock across the chest	मुटुको अनियमित धड्कन ठिक पार्ने काम
deficiency (n)	a lack of an essential quality or element	कमि
deficit (n)	the amount by which something, as a sum of money, falls short of the required or expected amount; shortage	कमि
deformity (n)	the state of being misshapen or disfigured	बिकृति
degeneration (n)	the process of losing function, or a decline from an original state	नराम्रो हुनु
degenerative (n)	undergoing a decline, as in function or nature, from a former or original state	नराम्रो बनाउने कुनै रोग
degenerative disc (n)	a condition characterized by a decline in the function of the discs in joints, esp. in the spine	जोर्नीको भित्रि भाग नराम्रो बनाउने रोग
degenerative joint disease (n)	a condition characterized by a decline in function of the joints, osteoarthritis	जोर्नीको अवस्था नराम्रो बनाउने रोग
degradation (n)	the act or process of decomposing or lowering by wear	नराम्रो हुनु
dehydrate (v)	to remove water from the body	निर्जलीकरण गर्नु
dehydration (n)	the condition that results from excessive loss of body water	निर्जलीकरण

English-Nepali Medical Glossary – D

Term	Definition	Nepali
delirium (n)	an acute, reversible organic mental disorder characterized by reduced ability to maintain attention	ध्यान केन्द्रित गर्न नसक्ने
deliver, give birth (v)	to assist in giving birth; to assist or aid in the birth of	जन्म दिनु
delivery room (n)	the location where a woman gives birth	बच्चा जन्माउने कोठा
delivery, childbirth (n)	the act of giving birth	बच्चाको जन्म हुने प्रक्रिया
delusion (n)	a false opinion or idea	भ्रम
dementia (n)	a mental disorder characterized by a general loss of intellectual abilities	बौद्धिकता हराउने एक मानासिक स्थिति
dental floss (n)	a strong waxed or unwaxed thread used to clean areas between the teeth	दाँतमा अड्केको बस्तु हटाउन प्रयोग गरीने धागो
dental hygiene (n)	a term used for maintaining teeth and the oral cavity by brushing, flossing, and visiting a dentist regularly	दाँतको सरसफाई
dental plaque (n)	a soft, thin film of food debris and other substances deposited on the teeth	दाँत माथिको पातलो झिल्ली
dentist (n)	a person whose profession is dentistry	दन्त चिकित्सक
dentistry (n)	the diagnosis, prevention, and treatment of diseases of the teeth and related structures	दन्त चिकित्सा
denture (n)	a set of artificial teeth	कृत्रिम दाँतहरुको पंक्ति
dependent (n)	contingent upon something or someone else	आश्रित
depersonalization (n)	alteration in the perception of the self so that the usual sense of one's own reality is lost	स्वयंलाई बुझ्ने कुरामा परिवर्तन हुने मानासिक अवस्था
depigmentation (n)	removal or loss of pigment	रंग हराउनु

English-Nepali Medical Glossary – D

Term	Definition	Nepali
depletion (n)	the act or process of emptying; removal of fluid, such as blood	कमि, रिक्तता
depolarization (n)	the process or act of neutralizing polarity	गैर-ध्रुवीकरण
depress (v)	to push downward or to create emotional depression	उदास हुनु
depression (n)	a condition of lowered spirits or sadness	उदासी
deprivation (n)	loss or absence of parts, organs, powers, or things that are needed	अभाव
dermatitis (n)	inflammation of the skin	छालाको सुजन
dermatologist (n)	a person whose profession is dermatology	छालाको चिकित्सक
dermatology (n)	the medical study of the physiology and pathology of the skin	त्वचा बिज्ञान
dermatosis (n)	any skin disease, especially one not characterized by inflammation	छालाको रोग
descending colon (n)	the third section of the large intestine that moves feces and waste downward towards the rectum	ठुलो आन्द्राको तलतिरको भाग
desensitization (n)	the act of rendering less sensitive or insensitive, as to light or pain; reduction of allergic reaction	कम सम्बेदनशील बनाउने कार्य
dessert (n)	any of various foods that are often high in fat and sugar, usually eaten after a meal	मिठाई
detection (n)	the act of finding something or a substance through experiments or observation	पहिचान
detergent (n)	a cleansing substance made from chemical compounds rather than from fats and lye	सफाई गर्न प्रयोग गरीने रसायन

English-Nepali Medical Glossary – D

Term	Definition	Nepali
detoxification (n)	the act or process of counteracting or destroying the toxic properties of a substance	बिष नास गर्ने कार्य
dextrose (n)	sugars found in animal and plant tissue and derived from starch; also see *carbohydrate*	जिबित कोषमा पाइने चिनी
diabetes (n)	a general term referring to disorders characterized by excessive urine discharge and persistent thirst; most commonly, it refers to a condition associated with high blood sugar	मधुमेह
diabetes management (n)	the control of blood sugar (blood glucose) levels by regular exercise, eating a healthy diet and taking medications as prescribed, if needed	मधुमेहको व्यवस्थापन
diabetic (adj)	of, relating to, or having diabetes	मधुमेह भएको
diabetic retinopathy (n)	a common complication of diabetes affecting the blood vessels in the retina (the thin membrane that covers the back of the eye); if untreated, it may lead to blindness; if diagnosed and treated promptly, blindness is usually preventable	आँखामा असर गर्ने मधुमेहको जटिलता
diagnosis (n)	the act or process of identifying or determining the nature of a disease through examination; also the result of this process	निदान

Term	Definition	Nepali
diagnosis related groups (DRGs) (n)	a system of classification for inpatient hospital services based on principal diagnosis, secondary diagnosis, surgical procedures, age, sex, and presence of complications; this system of classification is used as a financing mechanism to reimburse hospital and other providers for services rendered	डाईग्नोसीस रिलेटेड ग्रुप्स (डी.आर.जीस्)
diagnostic test (n)	any of various tests used to detect a disease or determine a patient's medical condition	नैदानिक परिक्षण
dialysis (n)	the separation of smaller molecules from larger molecules; this technique is commonly used to remove waste or toxins from the body in patients whose kidneys do not work well	डायलाईसीस
diameter (n)	length of a straight line passing through the center of a circle and connecting opposite points on its circumference	व्यास
diaper (n)	a folded piece of cloth or other absorbent material placed between a baby's legs and pinned at the waist	थाङ्नोको कट्टु
diaper rash (n)	a skin irritation or redness caused by excessive use of a diaper	थाङ्ने कट्टूले पाछेको घाउ
diaphragm (n)	a contraceptive used in family planning that blocks the opening to the uterus	महिलाले प्रयोग गर्ने एक परिबार नियोजनको साधन
diaphragm (n)	a muscular wall separating abdominal and thoracic cavities, which helps in breathing	पेट र छातिलाई अलग राख्ने मांशपेशी

English-Nepali Medical Glossary – D

Term	Definition	Nepali
diarrhea (n)	a condition of having feces that contains abnormally high levels of water	पखाला
diastole (n)	the period when the heart is relaxed and is filling with blood	मुटु फुकेर रगतले भरिएको अवस्था
diastolic (adj)	of, or pertaining to the diastole	मुटु फुकेर रगतले भरिएको अवस्थासँग सम्बन्धित
die (v)	to cease living; to expire	मर्नु
diet (n)	the usual food and drink of a person; a regulated selection of foods, esp. as prescribed for medical reasons	आहार
dietitian (n)	a person specializing in the study of diet and dieting as it relates to health and hygiene	आहार विशेषज्ञ
difficulty (n)	the condition or quality of being hard to do, achieve, or perform	कठिनाई
diffusion (n)	the process of becoming widely spread	फैलाव
digestion (n)	the primary bodily process by which food is decomposed into simple, absorbable substances used in proper body function	पाचन
digestive (adj)	pertaining to digestion	पाचन कार्य सँग सम्बन्धित
digestive system (n)	the system of organs in the body involved in digestion, including the large intestines, small intestines, and accessory glands, including salivary glands, liver, and pancreas	पाचन प्रणाली
dilation (n)	the condition in which an opening is enlarged or stretched beyond the normal dimensions; the act or process of enlarging or stretching	फुलाई, फैलाव

English-Nepali Medical Glossary – D

Term	Definition	Nepali
dilation and curettage (n)	a surgical procedure that expands the cervical canal of the uterus so that the surface lining of the uterus can be scraped	पाठेघरको भित्रि भाग खुर्कने कार्य
diminished (adj)	a condition of having been reduced or made smaller	कम
diphtheria (n)	an acute contagious disease caused by infection and characterized by difficulty in breathing, high fever, and weakness	भ्यागुते रोग
disability (n)	a disabled condition; incapacity; something that disables; handicap	विकलांगता
disable (v) (m)	to weaken or destroy the normal physical or mental abilities of; to incapacitate	निष्क्रिय हुनु
discharge (n)	something that is discharged, released, or emitted	श्राव, रस
discharge (v)	to relieve of a burden or of contents; to release, such as to discharge pus; to release from confinement, such as to discharge from a hospital	छोड्नु, मुक्त गर्नु, श्राव हुनु
discharge planning (v)	the comprehensive evaluation of a patient's health needs in order to arrange for appropriate care after discharge from an institutional clinical care setting	डिस्चार्ज प्लानिङ
discomfort (n)	an unpleasant or painful sensation; a condition of not feeling good associated with a specific situation	असुविधा
disease (n)	illness or sickness often characterized by typical patient problems (symptoms) and physical findings (signs)	रोग

English-Nepali Medical Glossary – D

Term	Definition	Nepali
disinfect (v)	to clean by removing all substances that may cause an infection	संक्रमणजन्य जिबाणुहरु नाश पार्नु
disinfectant (n)	an agent that removes harmful microorganisms; applied particularly to destroy harmful microorganisms on inanimate objects	संक्रमणजन्य जिबाणुहरु नाश गर्ने पदार्थ
disk (n)	a thin, flat, circular plate	कुनै गोलो पातलो बस्तु
dislocate (v)	to displace a limb or organ from the normal position, esp. to displace a bone from the socket or joint	विस्थापित गर्नु, उखाल्नु, फुत्काउनु
dislocated (adj)	pertaining to something that is displaced	विस्थापित, उखेलिएको, फुत्किएको
dislocation (n)	the displacement of any part, esp. of a bone	फुत्काउने काम
disorientation (n)	the loss of proper bearings, or a state of mental confusion as to time, place, or identity	असामन्जस्य
disoriented (adj)	not knowing one's position or location; confused	असामन्जस्यता
disseminate (v)	to scatter or distribute over a considerable area	प्रसार गर्नु
dissociation (n)	the act of separating or state of being separated	पृथकीकरण
dissolve (v)	to cause to disappear in a liquid; to break into parts	घोल्नु
distend (v)	to swell out or expand from or as if from internal pressure	फुलाउनु, फैलाउनु
distention (n)	the state of being distended or enlarged; the act of distending	फुलाउने कार्य, फैलाउने कार्य
distortion (n)	the state of being twisted or bent out of a natural or normal shape or position	बटार्ने कार्य

English-Nepali Medical Glossary – D

Term	Definition	Nepali
distribution (n)	specific location or arrangement of objects, or of continuing or successive events in space or time	वितरण
disturbance (n)	the act of breaking up or destroying the settled state of; a departure or divergence from that which is considered normal	अशान्ति
diuretic (adj)	tending to increase the discharge of urine	पिशाब खुलाउने औषधि सम्बन्धि
diuretic (n)	a drug or agent that increases the discharge of urine	पिशाब खुलाउने औषधि, मूत्रवर्धक
diurnal (adj)	occurring during the day	दिनको, दैनिक
diverticulitis (n)	inflammation of a diverticulum, especially inflammation of the small pockets in the wall of the colon which fill with fecal material	खोक्रो अंग बाट निस्केको थैली जस्तो भागको सुजन
diverticulum (n)	a pouch or sac branching out from a hollow organ or structure, such as the intestine	खोक्रो अंग बाट थैली जस्तो निस्कनु
dizziness (n)	the sensation or feeling of whirling or tendency to fall	रिङ्गटा लाग्नु
dizzy (adj)	having a whirling sensation or feeling a tendency to fall	रिङ्गटा
doctor (n)	person trained in the healing arts and licensed to practice, esp. a physician, surgeon, dentist, or veterinarian	चिकित्सक
doctor's office (n)	the location where a doctor works and meets patients	चिकित्सकको कार्यालय
document (n)	an original or official paper relied upon as the basis, proof or support of something	दस्तावेज

English-Nepali Medical Glossary – D

Term	Definition	Nepali
domestic violence (n)	the emotional or physical force used with the intention of hurting someone typically a family member, a spouse, boyfriend or girlfriend	घरेलु हिंसा
dominance (n)	the act of gaining or displaying control over someone or something else; esp. in genetics, a human trait or characteristic that is visible (as opposed to an invisible recessive trait)	प्रभुत्व
donor (n)	an individual person that supplies living tissue to be used in another body, such as a person who furnishes a blood transfusion	दाता
dosage (n)	determination and regulation of the size, frequency, and number of doses	मात्रा
dosage schedule (n)	a scheme set up to determine and regulate size, frequency, and number of doses	मात्रको तालिका
dose (n)	quantity to be administered at one time, such as a specified amount of medication	मात्रा
double vision (n)	seeing two images of an object when only one is present	एउटै बस्तुलाई दुईवटा देख्नु
double-blind (adj)	pertaining to a clinical trial or other experiment in which neither the subject nor the person administering treatment knows which treatment any particular subject is receiving	औषधि उपचार दिने र लिने दुबैलाई थाह नदिई गरिने परीक्षण
douche (v)	to clean or apply a medication by directing a stream or current of water against a part, esp. the vagina	धारा बहाएर शरीरको कुनै भागको सफाइ गर्नु

Term	Definition	Nepali
Down's Syndrome (n)	a congenital disorder characterized by moderate to severe mental retardation, a short flattened skull, and slanting eyes	डाउन्स सिन्ड्रोम
drain (v)	to remove or empty liquid, esp. to remove fluid from a wound or internal cavity	बहाउनु
drainage (n)	the withdrawal of fluids and discharges from a wound, sore or cavity	नाली
dressing (n)	the therapeutic materials applied to a wound	मलमपट्टि
drop (n) (m)	a minute quantity of a substance	थोपा
drop (v) (m)	to let something fall down	खसाउनु
drown (v)	to kill by submerging and suffocating in water or another liquid	डुब्नु
drowsy (adj)	dull with sleepiness; sluggish	निन्द्रा लाग्नु
drug addict (n)	a person addicted to a substance or drug	लागूऔषधको कुलतमा लागेको व्यक्ति
drug addiction (n)	the state of being addicted to a substance or drug	लागूऔषधको कुलत
drug formulary (n)	a listing of prescription medications that are preferred for use by a health plan and which will be dispensed through participating pharmacies to covered persons; this list is subject to periodic review and modification	औषधिहरुको सङ्ग्रह सुची
drug overdose (n)	an excessive dose, usually having harmful effects	बढीमात्रामा औषधि लिएको अवस्था
drugstore (n)	a store where prescriptions are filled and drugs and other articles are sold	औषधि पसल

English-Nepali Medical Glossary – D

Term	Definition	Nepali
drunk (adj)	intoxicated with alcohol to the point of impairment of physical and mental faculties	नसा लागेको
dry heat (n)	a condition where the temperature is high but the humidity of the air is low; little water vapor in the air	सुक्खा गर्मि
dry mouth (n)	the lack of moisture or saliva in the mouth	सुक्खा मुख
dry nose (n)	the lack of moisture or mucus in the nose	सुक्खा नाक
duct (n)	a passage with well-defined walls, especially a tube for the passage of excretions or secretions	नली
duodenal ulcer (n)	an inflammatory lesion on the first section of the small intestine	सानो आन्द्राको माथिल्लो भागको घाउ
duodenum (n)	first or proximal portion of the small intestine, extending from the pylorus to the jejunum	सानो आन्द्राको माथिल्लो भाग
dura mater (n)	outermost, toughest section of membrane covering the brain and spinal cord	गिदीलाई ढाक्ने बाहिरी कडा झिल्ली
Durable Medical Equipment (DME) (n)	equipment, which can stand repeated use, that is primarily and customarily used to serve a medical purpose, generally is not useful to a person in the absence of illness or injury, and is appropriate for use at home; examples of durable medical equipment include hospital beds, wheelchairs, and oxygen equipment	टिकाउ चिकित्सा उपकरण (डी.एम.इ.)
duration (n)	continuance or persistence in time; period of time during which something exists or persists	अवधि

Term	Definition	Nepali
dust mite (n)	a very small insect that lives in house dust and commonly causes an allergic reaction	धुलोमा बस्ने एक प्रकारको घुन
dysentery (n)	any of various disorders marked by inflammation of the intestines, especially of the colon, and attended by pain in the abdomen, and stools containing blood and mucus	आऊँ
dysfunction (n)	disturbance, impairment, or abnormality of the functioning of an organ	खराब हुनु
dyslexia (n)	impairment of the ability to read	पढ्ने क्षमता कमजोर हुनु
dyspepsia (n)	disturbed digestion; indigestion	अपच
dysphasia (n)	impairment of speech due to brain injury	बोल्ने क्षमता कमजोर हुनु
dystrophy (n)	any disorder arising from defective or faulty nutrition, esp. muscular dystrophy	सुक्नु, आकार घट्नु

English-Nepali Medical Glossary – E

Term	Definition	Nepali
ear (n)	an organ of hearing, responsible, in general, for maintaining balance as well as sensing sound, and divided in humans into the external ear, the middle ear, and the internal ear	कान
ear bone (n)	one of three bones (the malleus, incus, or stapes) in the ear that assist in hearing	कानको हड्डी
ear canal (n)	the section of the ear leading to the middle ear	कानको नली
ear drops (n)	medicine administered directly into the ear, usually for healing an earache or to dissolve wax	कानमा हाल्ने औषधि
ear drum (n)	a membrane that separates the outer section of the ear from the middle and internal sections of the ear	कानको झिल्ली
ear infection (n)	an infection of the ear, usually causing inflammation and pain	कानको सङ्क्रमण
ear wax (n)	the wax-like secretions of certain glands lining the canal of the outer ear	कानेगुजी
ear, nose, and throat (n)	a branch of medicine studying the ears, nose, and throat	नाक, कान, घाँटी
ear, nose, and throat specialist (n)	a physician who specializes in the branch of medicine that combines treatment of the ear, nose, and throat	नाक, कान, घाँटी बिशेषज्ञ
earache (n)	an ache or pain in the ear	कान दुख्ने
earlobe (n)	the fleshy bottom portion of the external ear	कानको लोती
echocardiography (n)	a diagnostic technique utilizing ultrasound to visualize the internal structure of the heart	इकोकार्डियोग्राफी, मुटुको बनावट अवलोकन गर्ने काम

English-Nepali Medical Glossary – E

Term	Definition	Nepali
eclampsia (n)	convulsions and coma occurring in a pregnant woman, associated with preeclampsia, i.e., hypertension and edema	गर्भवती महिलामा हुने बेहोसी र कम्पन
ectopic pregnancy (n)	the development of a fetus outside the uterus	पाठेघर बाहिर गर्भ रहनु
eczema (n)	a noncontiguous inflammation of the skin, marked mainly by redness, itching, and the outbreak of lesions that discharge matter and become encrusted and scaly	एक प्रकारको चिलाउने चर्मरोग
edema (n)	an excessive accumulation of fluid in tissue caused by diseases of the heart, kidney, liver, and veins	पानी भरिएर सुन्निने
effect (n)	result produced by an action	असर
effective (adj)	producing the intended result	प्रभावकारी
effusion (n)	escape of fluid into a part of tissue	बहाव
eggs (n)	1. the thin-shelled embryo of any bird, high in protein and cholesterol, and eaten alone or added to many foods including baked foods, breads, pasta, and packaged foods; 2. human egg cell	अण्डाहरु
ejaculation (n)	a sudden act of expulsion; the sexual climax or orgasm in a male causing the release of semen	स्खलन
eject (v)	to throw out forcefully; to expel	बलपूर्वक निकाल्नु
elastic (adj)	capable of resisting and recovering from stretching, compression, or distortion applied by force	लचकदार
elbow (n)	the joint or bend of the arm between the forearm and the upper arm	कुहिनो

English-Nepali Medical Glossary – E

Term	Definition	Nepali
elective (n)	subject to the choice or decision of the patient or physician; applied to procedures that are advantageous to the patient but not urgent	वैकल्पिक
electric stimulation (n)	transcutaneous electric nerve stimulation (TENS); therapy to reduce pain and restore muscle action	बिद्युतिय उत्तेजना
electrocardiogram (n)	a graph created by monitoring the electrical action of the heart; it is used to diagnose heart disease	मुटुको बिद्युतिय गतिविधिको रेखा-चित्र
electrocardiograph (n)	an instrument used to record the potential of the electric currents that traverse the heart and initiate its contraction	मुटुको बिद्युतिय गतिविधिको रेखा-चित्र लिने यन्त्र
electroencephalography (n)	the recording of the electric currents developed in the brain, by means of electrodes applied to the scalp, to the surface of the brain, or placed within the substance of the brain; it is commonly used to diagnose seizures	दिमागको बिद्युतिय गतिविधिको रेखा-चित्र लिने कार्य
electrolyte (n)	substance that dissociates into ions when in a solution, and is capable of conducting electricity	इलेक्ट्रोलाइट
electromyelogram (n)	a graphic recording of muscle action	मांसपेशीको गतिविधिको रेखा-चित्र
elevator (n)	a platform or enclosure raised and lowered in a vertical shaft to transport things or people	लिफ्ट
elimination (n)	the act of removing; the excretion of waste from the body	निष्कासन, त्याग

Term	Definition	Nepali
elisa test (n)	enzyme-linked immunosorbent assay; a sensitive diagnostic test for measuring the amount of a substance (e.g., used in HIV testing)	एड्सको एक नैदानिक परिक्षण
embolism (n)	sudden blocking of an artery by a clot or foreign material	धमनीमा अचानक हुने रोकावट
embryo (n)	the developing baby in the uterus from about two weeks after fertilization to the end of the seventh or eighth week	भ्रुण
emergency (n)	an unexpected situation or sudden occurrence of a serious and urgent nature, usually life threatening, that demands immediate action	आपतकालीन अवस्था
emergency room (n)	the section of the hospital where emergency cases are treated	आपतकालीन कक्ष
emergency services (n)	health services that are required for the alleviation of severe pain or immediate diagnosis and treatment of unforeseen medical conditions, which if not immediately diagnosed and treated, could lead to disability or death	आपतकालीन सेवाहरु
emesis (n)	vomiting; an act of vomiting	बान्ता
emetic (adj)	an agent that causes vomiting	बान्ता गराउने बस्तु
emollient (n)	an agent that softens or soothes	नरम बनाउने वा आराम दिने बस्तु
emotion (n)	a complex and usually strong feeling or response, such as love or fear	भावना
emotional (adj)	of, or pertaining to emotion	भावुक

English-Nepali Medical Glossary – E

Term	Definition	Nepali
emphysema (n)	an accumulation of air in tissues or organs; applied especially to such a condition of the lungs	वातस्फीति, फोक्सोमा हावा अड्किएको अवस्था
empiric (adj)	depending upon experience or observation alone, without using a scientific method or theory	अनुभवसिद्ध
enamel (n)	the hard substance covering the exposed portion of a tooth	दाँतको खोल
encephalitis (n)	inflammation of the brain	इन्सेफलाइटिस, दिमागको सुजन
encounter (n)	a medically related service or visit rendered by a provider (or providers) to a beneficiary who is enrolled in a health plan on a specific date of service; it includes, but is not limited to, all services for which the health plan contractor incurred any financial liability	चिकित्सा सम्बद्ध एक सेवा
endemic (adj)	of, or pertaining to a disease present or usually prevalent in a population or geographical area at all times	खास जाति वा क्षेत्रमा सिमित रोग
endocrine system (n)	pertaining to the functioning and regulation of glands that secrete hormones throughout the body	अन्त:श्राव प्रणाली
endocrinologist (n)	a person whose profession is to study the physiology of the endocrine glands	एंडोक्राइनोलॉजिस्ट, अन्त:श्राव रोग विशेषज्ञ
endometriosis (n)	a condition in which endometrial-like tissue is found in the pelvic region	इन्डोमेट्रीओसीस
endometrium (n)	the membrane lining the uterus	पाठेघरको भित्रि झिल्ली
endoscope (n)	an instrument for examining the interior of a bodily canal or hollow organ	खोक्रो अंगको अवलोकन गर्ने यन्त्र

English-Nepali Medical Glossary – E

Term	Definition	Nepali
endoscopy(n)	visual inspection of any cavity of the body by using an endoscope	खोक्रो अंगको अवलोकन
endotrachael intubation (n)	a surgical procedure that places a tube directly into the airway by way of the trachea to assist breathing	श्वासनलीमा नली राख्ने कार्य
endotracheal tube (n)	a tube inserted into the trachea to assist breathing	श्वासनलीमा राखिने नली
enema (n)	an injection of liquid into the rectum through the anus for cleansing, as a laxative, or for other therapeutic purposes	एनिमा
energetic (adj)	exhibiting energy; strenuous; operating with force, vigor, or effect	ऊर्जावान
energy (n)	the element a body requires to grow, develop, and work properly	ऊर्जा
enrollee (n)	one who has entered a program	भर्ना भएको व्यक्ति
environment (n)	sum total of all the conditions and elements which make up the surroundings of and influence the development and actions of an individual	वातावरण
enzyme (n)	a protein molecule that helps chemical reactions of other substances without itself being destroyed or altered upon completion of the reactions	इन्जाइम
epidemic (adj)	of, or pertaining to a disease that effects many people at the same time in the same geographic area	महामारी
epidemiological (adj)	relating to, or involving the study of how diseases develop, spread, and affect populations	महामारी विज्ञान सम्बन्धि

English-Nepali Medical Glossary – E

Term	Definition	Nepali
epidermal (adj)	of, or pertaining to, or resembling the outer, protective surface of skin, esp. a type of injection made into the skin	छालाको बाहिरी सतह सँग सम्बन्धित
epidural (adj)	situated upon or outside the dura mater	मेरुदण्डको तल्लो छेउको एक भाग
epiglottis (n)	a small piece of cartilage that prevents food from entering the lungs when swallowing by covering the windpipe	उपकण्ठ
epilepsy (n)	a disorder characterized by recurring attacks of motor, sensory, or psychic malfunction with or without unconsciousness or convulsive movements	छारे रोग
epiphyseal (adj)	pertaining to or of the nature of a section of a bone, often an end of a long bone, that initially develops separated from the main portion by cartilage	एपिफाईसीयल
episiotomy (n)	surgical incision into the region between the vagina and anus to prevent traumatic tearing during delivery of a baby	योनी र मलद्वारको बिचमा चिर्ने कार्य
episode (n)	a noteworthy happening or series of happenings occurring in the course of continuous events, such as an episode of illness; a separate but related incident	प्रकरण
epithelial (adj)	of, or pertaining to the epithelium	सतहमा हुने कोषहरुको एक तह सँग सम्बन्धित
epithelium (n)	the layer of cells that form the surface lining of the mouth, digestive tract, and other mucous surfaces	सतहमा हुने कोषहरुको एक तह

English-Nepali Medical Glossary – E

Term	Definition	Nepali
equivalent (n)	having the same value; neutralizing or counterbalancing	बराबर
erection (n)	condition of being made rigid and elevated, esp. the enlargement of the penis when aroused	लिङ्गको उत्तेजना
erosion (n)	the destruction of the surface of a tissue, material, or structure	कटान, क्षय
eruption (n)	act of breaking out, appearing, or becoming visible, as eruption of the teeth	बिस्फोट
erythema (n)	an area of skin which is red in color	छालाको बिबिरा
esophagitis (n)	inflammation of the esophagus or throat	अन्ननलीको सुजन
esophagus (n)	a muscular membranous tube for the passage of food from the mouth to the stomach	अन्ननली
estrogen (n)	any of several steroid hormones produced chiefly by the ovary and responsible for promoting the development and maintenance of female secondary sex characteristics, such as breasts	इस्ट्रोजेन
etiology (n)	study of the causes of disease	रोगको कारणको अध्ययन
euphoria (n)	an exaggerated feeling of physical and mental well-being, especially when not justified by external reality	उल्लास
eustachian tube (n)	a bony and cartilaginous tube connecting the ear with the throat	कानलाई गलासँग जोड्ने नली
evacuation (n)	an emptying, esp. of the bowels	खालि गर्ने कार्य
evaluation (n)	the act or result of ascertaining or fixing the value or worth of; the act or result of examining or judging carefully	मूल्याङ्कन

English-Nepali Medical Glossary – E

Term	Definition	Nepali
event monitor (n)	portable instrument used to monitor heart function	इभेन्ट मनिटर
evolution (n)	process of development in which an organ or organism becomes more complex or changes due to pressures caused by the environment	विकासक्रम
exacerbation (n)	increase in the severity of a disease or its symptoms	रोगले चाप्नु
exam (n) (m)	an examination or the act of observing, analyzing, questioning, and testing the state or condition of a person	परीक्षा
exam room (n)	the location where a doctor examines a patient	परीक्षा कोठा
excessive (adj)	exceeding the usual, proper, or normal quantity; more than necessary	अत्याधिक
excrete (v)	to eliminate waste from the blood, tissues, or organs	निष्कासन गर्नु
excretion (n)	the act, process, or function of eliminating waste from blood, tissue, or organs	निष्कासन
exercise (n)	activity that requires physical or mental exertion, esp. when performed to develop or maintain fitness or good health	व्यायाम
exercise tolerance test (n)	a method of measuring a person's level of physical condition	व्यायाम सहनसिलता परिक्षण
exfoliation (n)	a falling off in scales or layers, esp. the loss of skin	छालाको पत्र झर्नु
exhale (v)	to breathe out	श्वास फाल्नु
exit (n) (m)	a passage or way out	प्रस्थान

English-Nepali Medical Glossary – E

Term	Definition	Nepali
expectorant (n)	a drug/substance that promotes the ejection, by spitting, of mucus or other fluids from the lungs and throat	कफ निकाल्ने औषधि
experimental (adj) (m)	of, or pertaining to, or based upon a test procedure, idea or activity	प्रयोगात्मक
expiration (n)	the act of breathing out, or expelling air from the lungs	श्वास फाल्ने कार्य
exploratory surgery (n)	a surgical procedure used to investigate systematically a part of the body for the purpose of diagnosis	नैदानिक शल्यक्रिया
extend (v)	to straighten a leg or an arm	सिधा पार्नु
external use (n)	generally used in describing products such as ointments, salves, eye or ear drops that are not to be ingested and are for 'external use'	बाहिरी प्रयोगका लागि मात्र
extract (v)	to separate a substance from something, esp. the removal of a desired substance from a plant or animal in order to prepare a drug	सारतत्व निकाल्नु
extraction (n)	the process or act of pulling or drawing out	झिक्ने वा निकाल्ने कार्य
extreme (adj)	as far away as possible from the center, the beginning or the average; of the highest degree or intensity	अत्याधिक, टाढा
extremity (n)	a limb; an arm or leg; sometimes applied specifically to a hand or foot	हातखुट्टा
eye (n)	an organ that allows humans to see and sense light	आँखा
eye chart (n)	an instrument used to determine the quality of someone's vision	दृष्टि जाँच तालिका
eye drops (n)	a liquid medicine placed on the surface of the eye	आँखामा राखिने औषधि

English-Nepali Medical Glossary – E

Term	Definition	Nepali
eye exam (n)	a procedure where the physician studies the patient's eyes to detect any disease or vision problems	आँखाको परिक्षण
eye patch (n)	a protective covering for the eye	आँखा छोप्ने टालो
eye strain (n)	over use of the muscles surrounding the eye characterized by pain in the eyes, tears, headache, or dizziness	आँखा दुख्नु
eyeball (n)	the eye itself; the ball-shaped portion of the eye	आँखाको नानी
eyebrows (n)	the bony ridge extending over the eye; the arch of short hairs covering this ridge	आँखीभौँ
eyelash (n)	one of a row of short hairs at the edge of the eyelid	परेलाको रौँ
eyelid (n)	either of two folds of skin and muscle that can be closed over an eye	परेला

Term	Definition	Nepali
face (n)	the surface of the front of the head from the top of the forehead to the base of the chin and from ear to ear	अनुहार
face-lift operation (n)	plastic surgery for tightening facial tissues and improving the appearance of facial skin	अनुहारको छाला राम्रो देखाउनको लागि गरीने शल्यक्रिया
facial (adj)	of, or pertaining to the face	अनुहारको
faint (v) (m)	to suddenly lose strength or vigor; to fall unconscious	मुर्छा पर्नु
faith (n)	firm and devoted adherence, as to a person, idea, or thing	आस्था
fallopian tube (n)	either of a pair of slender ducts that connect the uterus to the ovaries in the female reproductive system	डिम्बबाहिनी नली
family (n)	a group of persons sharing common ancestry	परिवार
family doctor (n)	a physician who does not specialize in a particular area but treats a variety of medical problems, usually serving a family	परिवारको चिकित्सक
family nurse practitioner (n)	a nurse who is licensed to treat people of any age	परिवारको नर्स
family planning (n)	planning of the number of one's children through birth-control techniques	परिवार नियोजन
farsighted (n)	able to see objects better from a distance than from short range	दुरदृष्टि
fast (v) (m)	to eat very little, nothing, or only select foods	निराहार बस्नु

English-Nepali Medical Glossary – F

Term	Definition	Nepali
fast foods (n)	any of various foods high in cholesterol, oils, and fats, including hamburgers, hotdogs, french fries, and pizza, and purchased at a grocery store or restaurant	तुरुन्तै तयार हुने खाना
fat (n)	the main storage and source of energy in humans; a high energy nutrient found in butter, lard, grease, and oil, also found at high levels in meat, desserts, cheese, cream, and milk	बोसो
fatal (adj)	causing death, deadly; mortal; lethal	घातक
fatigue (n)	a feeling of tiredness following exercise or strenuous activities	थकान
feces (n)	the substance discharged from the intestines, consisting of bacteria, cells, secretions (chiefly of the liver), and a small amount of undigested food	दिशा
federal (n)	belonging to the central government of the United States	संघिय
Federal Financial Participation (n)	federal expenditures provided to match proper State expenditures made under State approved plans	फेडेरल फाइनान्सियल पार्टीसिपेसन
Federal Poverty Level (n)	poverty guidelines of the federal poverty measure. They are issued each year in the Federal Register by the Department of Health and Human Services (HHS). The guidelines are a simplification of the poverty thresholds for use for administrative purposes — for instance, determining financial eligibility for certain federal programs	फेडेरल पोभर्टी लेभल

Term	Definition	Nepali
federally funded (n)	supported by monies from the Federal government	संघीय लगानीको
feedback (n)	the return of information about the result of a process, idea or activity	पृष्ठपोषण
fee-for-service (n)	a method of reimbursement based on payment for specific services rendered to an enrollee. Payment may be made by an insurance carrier. Fee-for-service is the traditional method of reimbursement used by physicians and almost always occurs retrospectively (i.e. after the service has been rendered)	सेवा शुल्क
femur (n)	the bone in the leg that extends from the hip to the knee; the femur constitutes the upper leg, that part of the leg above the knee and is the largest bone in the human body	तिघ्राको हड्डी
fertile (adj)	capable of reproducing	प्रजनन् क्षमता भएको
fertility (n)	the capacity to have a baby or to become pregnant	प्रजनन् क्षमता
fester (v)	to generate pus	पिप भरिएर पाक्नु, कुहिनु
fetal heart tone (n)	the heart beat of a fetus	भ्रूणको मुटुको धड्कन
fetal surgery (n)	any procedure that involves surgery on a fetus	भ्रूणको शल्यक्रिया
fetus (n)	the unborn young of a human from the eighth week of pregnancy until birth	भ्रुण
fever (n)	abnormally high body temperature, usually associated with illness	ज्वरो

English-Nepali Medical Glossary – F

Term	Definition	Nepali
fiber (n) (m)	a slender, long structure; any of the elongated cells of muscle tissue; any of the filaments making up connective tissue	रेशा
fiber (n) (m)	an important nutrient found in fruits, cereals, and grains	रेशा
fibroid (n)	resembling or composed of fibrous tissue	रेशेदार
fibroid tumor (n)	a benign tumor of smooth muscle, esp. in the uterus	रेशेदार क्यान्सर
fibrous (adj)	of, pertaining to, or resembling fiber	रेशायुक्त
fibula (n)	the outer and smaller of two bones of the leg between the knee and ankle	खुट्टाको नलीहाड
file (n)	a collection of information organized and easily retrievable, esp. a patient's history	फाइल
filling (n)	something used to fill a space, cavity, or container, such as a tooth filling	खालि ठाउँ भर्न प्रयोग गरीने बस्तु
filtration (n)	passage of a liquid through a filter, accomplished by gravity, pressure, or vacuum suction	छनाई
finger (n)	one of the five digits of the hand, esp. one other than the thumb	औंला
fingernail (n)	a thin, horny, transparent plate covering the surface of the tip of each finger	औंलाको नङ
fingerprint (n)	the pattern on a surface left by the finger and used in identification	औठाछाप
fingertips (n)	the end or distal section of the finger	औंलाको टुप्पो
fire extinguisher (n)	a portable or wheeled apparatus used for putting out small fires; it ejects extinguishing chemicals	अग्नि नियन्त्रक

English-Nepali Medical Glossary – F

Term	Definition	Nepali
first aid (n)	emergency treatment administered to injured or sick persons before professional medical care is available	प्राथमिक उपचार
fissure (n)	any cleft or groove, normal or otherwise, such as a fold in the cerebral cortex, skin, or mucous membrane	खोल्सो, चिरा
fistula (n)	an abnormal passage or communication, usually between two internal organs, or leading from an internal organ to the surface of the body	नालव्रण, साँगुरो मुख भएको घाऊ
fixation (n) (m)	he act or operation of holding, suturing, or fastening in a fixed position	निश्चित आसनमा बाध्ने वा सिउने काम
flaccid (adj)	weak, lax, and soft	चाउरी परेको, झोल्लिएको
flare-up (n)	a sudden outburst or intensification	अचानक बिष्फोट हुनु, भड्किनु
flatulence (n)	presence of excessive amounts of air or gases in the stomach or intestine, leading to enlarging of the organs	पेट फुल्नु, बायु भरिनु
fleshy (adj)	similar or related to the soft tissue of the body, skin, or flesh; having a juicy or pulpy feeling	मांसल
floaters (n)	black spots in front of the eyes caused by debris in the fluid inside the eye	आँखा अगाडीको कालो थोप्ला
floss (n)	a piece of waxed or unwaxed string used to remove plaque from below the gums and between the teeth	दाँत सफा गर्नु

English-Nepali Medical Glossary – F

Term	Definition	Nepali
flu (n)	influenza; an acute infectious disease causing inflammation of the respiratory tract, fever, muscular pain, and irritation in the digestive system	इन्फ्लुएन्जा
fluoride (n)	a chemical compound used by dentists to help prevent tooth decay and disease	फ्लोराइड
fluoroscopy (n)	a process using x-rays that allows continuous viewing of the internal structure of a human	फ्लुरोस्कोपी
flush (v) (m)	to become red, esp. the skin on the face, usually from certain diseases, ingestion of certain drugs or other substances, heat, emotional factors, or physical exertion	अनुहार रातो हुनु
flutter (n)	a disturbance of normal heart rhythm	मुटुको असामान्य स्पन्दन
foam (n)	a mass of gas bubbles, esp. a light, bubbly gas and liquid mass formed by shaking a liquid containing certain soaps or detergents	फिंज
follow-up (n)	the act or process of meeting again with a physician to reassess a person's health	पछि लाग्नु
fontanelle (n)	the soft portion of a baby's skull	बच्चाको खोपडीको नरम भाग
Food and Drug Administration (n)	a federal consumer protection agency; its mission is to promote and protect public health by helping safe and effective products reach the market in a timely way, and monitoring products for continued safety after they are in use	फुड एण्ड ड्रग एडमिनिस्ट्रेसन

English-Nepali Medical Glossary – F

Term	Definition	Nepali
Food Guide Pyramid (n)	a graphic representation of guidelines developed to help people choose what to eat and how much to eat from the five basic food groups in order to get needed nutrients	फुड गाइड पिरामिड
food poisoning (n)	poisoning or illness caused by eating food contaminated by natural toxins or bacteria	विषाक्त भोजन
foot (n)	the lower part of the leg that is in direct contact with the ground in standing or walking	पैताला
forceps (n)	an instrument like a pair of tongs, used for grasping, manipulating, or extracting	चिम्टा
forearm (n)	the part of the arm between the elbow and the hand	पाखुरा
forehead (n)	the part of the head or face between the eyebrows and the normal hairline	निधार
foreskin (n)	the excess of skin covering the end of the penis	लिङ्गको अगाडिको भाग ढाक्ने छाला
fraction (n)	a small part; bit; a substance separated from another	अंश
fracture (n)	a break or rupture in a bone	भाँचीएको
freckle (n)	a small spot of coloring in the skin, often brought out by the sun	पोतो, चाँयाँ
frequency (n) (m)	number of occurrences of a periodic or recurrent process per unit of time	आवृत्ति, नित्यता
fried food (n)	any of various foods cooked in oil and high in fats and cholesterol, including french fries, fried chicken, or fried fish	तारिएको खाना
fright (n)	sudden, intense fear, as of something immediately threatening, alarming, or strange	डर

English-Nepali Medical Glossary – F

Term	Definition	Nepali
frighten (v)	to make afraid; to alarm	डराउनु
front desk (n)	a location in a building used to greet people as they enter, manned/serviced by a desk clerk	स्वागत डेस्क
frostbite (n)	local tissue destruction resulting from freezing, esp. damaged skin of the fingers and toes	हिउँले खाएको
frozen shoulder (n)	a shoulder that cannot be moved	चलाउन नसकिने काँध
fruit (n)	a sweet and fleshy part of a plant, served as food, such as oranges, apples, grapes, plums, and bananas	फल
fruit juices (n)	any of various beverages made from the liquid of a fruit	फलको रस
function (n) (m)	the special, normal, or proper activity of an organ or part	कार्य
fundamental (adj)	of, or pertaining to a base or foundation, esp. the foundation of an idea	आधारभूत
funeral home (n)	an establishment in which the dead are prepared for burial or cremation, and in which wakes and funerals may be held	अन्तिम संस्कार भवन
fungicide (n)	an agent that destroys fungi	ढुसीनाशक
fungus (n)	general term used to denote a group of cellular organisms including mushrooms, yeasts, rusts, molds, smuts, etc.	ढुसी

English-Nepali Medical Glossary – G

Term	Definition	Nepali
gait (n)	manner or style of walking	हिंडाई
gallbladder (n)	a small pear-shaped muscular sac located under the liver, in which bile secreted by the liver is stored	पित्तथैली
gallstone (n)	a small, hard mass formed in the gallbladder or in a bile duct	पित्तको पत्थरी
gallstone disease (n)	stones the size of pebbles within the gallbladder, the pear-shaped sac beneath the liver that stores the bile secreted by the liver, or in the ducts that lead from the gallbladder to the intestine. Gallstones are a frequent cause of abdominal pain. They often trigger inflammation and infection of the gallbladder and the pancreas	पित्तथैलीको पत्थरी
ganglion (n)	a group of nerve cells found outside of the brain or spinal cord	स्नायुकोषहरुको समुह, नाड़ीग्रन्थि
gangrene (n)	the death and decay of tissue, usually caused by infection, injury, or lack of blood supply to the tissue	कुहिनु
gargle (v)	to force exhaled air through a liquid held in the back of the mouth in order to cleanse or medicate the mouth or throat	कुल्ला गर्नु
gas (n)	the state of matter distinguished from solid and liquid states by very low density (e.g., air that passes through the intestine, air inhaled for anesthesia) and the ability to diffuse readily	ग्यास, बायु
gastric (adj)	of, or pertaining to the stomach	पेटको
gastric bleeding (n)	bleeding in the stomach	पेटमा भएको रक्तश्राव

English-Nepali Medical Glossary – G

Term	Definition	Nepali
gastric juice (n)	secretions in the stomach that assist in digestion	पेटमा हुने पाचन रस
gastric ulcer (n)	an ulcer located in the stomach	पेटको घाऊ
gastritis (n)	inflammation of the stomach	पेटको सुजन
gastroenteritis (n)	an acute inflammation of the lining of the stomach and intestines, characterized by nausea, diarrhea, abdominal pain, and weakness, which has various causes, including food poisoning and infection	आन्द्राभुँडीको सुजन
gastroenterologist (n)	person who specializes in diseases of the digestive tract	पेटरोग विशेषज्ञ
Gastroesophageal Reflux Disease (GERD) (n)	a condition wherein acidic stomach contents regurgitate or back up (reflux) into the esophagus, causing inflammation and damage to the esophagus; this frequently causes heartburn because of irritation of the esophagus by stomach acid	ग्यास्ट्रोइसोफेजिएल रिफ्लक्स डिजिज (जी.ए.आर.डी.)
gastrointestinal (adj)	of, or pertaining to, or communication with the stomach and intestine	आन्द्राभुँडीको
gatekeeper (n)	the term used in a managed care plan to refer to the physician who has primary responsibility for providing basic medical services and coordinating a patient's medical care and referrals; in order for a patient to receive specialty referrals or a hospital admission, the gatekeeper must typically authorize it, unless there is an emergency	द्वारपाल

English-Nepali Medical Glossary – G

Term	Definition	Nepali
gauze (n)	a thin, transparent fabric with a loose open weave, used for covering wounds	पट्टि
gene (n)	a functional hereditary unit that occupies a fixed location on a chromosome, has a specific influence on the phenotype, and is capable of mutating	जीन
general anesthesia (n)	the use of drugs to cause a person to lose all sense of feeling, thus enabling painless surgery	बेहोस पार्ने औषधि
general practitioner (n)	a physician who does not specialize in a particular area but treats a variety of medical problems	साधारण चिकित्सक
genetic (adj)	of, or pertaining to genes, reproduction, or to birth	आनुवंशिक
genetic counseling (n)	the counseling of prospective parents on the probabilities of inherited diseases occurring in offspring and on the diagnosis and treatment of such diseases	आनुवंशिक परामर्श
genetic factors (n)	biological information (genes, characteristics) that parents pass on to their children	आनुवंशिक कारण
genetic tendency (n)	susceptibility to a particular disease due to genetics	आनुवंशिक प्रवृत्ति
genital (adj)	of, or relating to reproduction; of, or pertaining to the genitalia	जनेन्द्रीयको
genitalia (n)	the reproductive organs, esp. the external sexual organs	जनेन्द्रीय
geriatric (n)	having to do with senior citizens	बुढ्यौली
germ (n) (m)	pathogenic microorganism; something that may serve as the basis of further growth or development	किटाणु

English-Nepali Medical Glossary – G

Term	Definition	Nepali
German Measles (n)	a mild, contagious, eruptive disease with widespread pink rash caused by a virus and capable of causing defects in infants born to mothers infected during the first three months of pregnancy (i.e., rubella)	जर्मन दादुरा
gestation (n)	period of development of the young, from the time of fertilization of the ovum until birth	गर्भावधि
gestational diabetes (n)	a specific form of diabetes caused by pregnancy	गर्भावधिको मधुमेह
gingivitis (n)	inflammation of the gums	गिंजा सुन्निनु
give a shot (v)	to inject medicine under a person's skin	सूई हाल्नु
gland (n)	an organ that extracts specific substances from the blood and concentrates or alters them for subsequent secretion	ग्रन्थी
glandular (adj)	of, or pertaining to, or resembling a gland or the activities of a gland	ग्रन्थिको
glans penis (n)	the end of the penis	लिङ्गको टुप्पो
glasses (eye) (n)	a pair of lenses mounted in a light frame, used to correct poor vision or to protect the eyes	चस्मा
glaucoma (n)	a disease of the eye characterized by an increase in pressure in the eye, which causes defects in vision	ग्लोकोमा, मोतिबिन्दु
glottis (n)	the space between the vocal chords at the upper part of the larynx or voice box	श्वासनलीको मुख
glucometer (n)	a device that measures the amount of sugar in a human's blood	ग्लुकोज मापक यन्त्र

Term	Definition	Nepali
glucose (n)	sugar found in certain foods, especially fruits, and in the normal blood of all animals; a major source of energy for humans, also see *carbohydrate*	ग्लुकोज
gluten (n)	protein of wheat and other grains	ग्लुटेन
goiter (n)	a chronic enlargement of the thyroid gland, visible as swelling at the front of the neck, associated with iodine deficiency	गलगाँड
gonad (n)	an organ involved in reproduction, i.e., the testis or ovaries	जननग्रंथि
gonorrhea (n)	sexually transmitted infection; male may experience pain and discharge from the penis; female may be asymptomatic or have vaginal discharge	गोनेरिया
gout (n)	a disturbance of the metabolic system occurring predominantly in males, characterized by painful inflammation of the joints, esp. of the feet and hands	बातरोग
gown (hospital) (n)	a loose garment worn by patients in the hospital	गाउन (अस्पतालको)
gradual (adj)	taking place by a series of small changes over a long period; not sudden	बिस्तारै
grains (n)	any of various small hard seeds used in making bread or cereal and high in fiber and carbohydrates	अनाज
Graves Disease (n)	a disease causing a toxic goiter	घातक गलगाँड
gravidity (n)	pregnancy; the condition of being pregnant, without regard to the outcome	गर्भावस्था

Term	Definition	Nepali
grievance (n)	1) a written request by a provider for a health plan to review an adverse action decision, or policy issued by the health plan which has a direct effect on the provider; and 2) a written request by a member for a health plan to review an action or decision by the health plan or one of its providers	शिकायत, गुनासो
groin (n)	the area of the body found between the legs and at the junction between the trunk and legs, including the external genitals	काप
guardian (n)	person charged with the care of the person or property of another	अभिभावक
gums (n)	that part of the lining of the oral cavity (oral mucosa) that surrounds the base of the teeth generally red or pink in color; it may be the site of injury, inflammation, bleeding or infection; often a concern if the gums are receding, starting to cover less and less of a tooth or a series of teeth	गिंजा
gun shot wound (n)	any injury resulting from a bullet	गोलीले बनाएको घाउ
gynecological (adj)	of, or pertaining to gynecology	स्त्रीरोग सम्बन्धी
gynecology (n)	the medical science of disease, reproductive physiology, and endocrinology in women	स्त्रीरोग विज्ञान
gynocologist (n)	a person who studies diseases, disorders, and physiology of the female reproductive organs	स्त्रीरोग विशेषज्ञ

English-Nepali Medical Glossary – H

Term	Definition	Nepali
habitual (adj)	the nature of a habit; according to habit; something done repeatedly without thinking	अभ्यस्त
Haemophilus Influenza Type B (HiB) (n)	a bacteria capable of causing a range of diseases including ear infections, cellulitis (soft tissue infection), upper respiratory infections, pneumonia, and such serious "invasive" infections as meningitis with potential brain damage and epiglottitis with airway obstruction; more than 90% of all HIB infections occur in children 5 years of age or less; the peak attack rate is at 6-12 months of age	हेमोफिलस इन्फ्लुएन्जा टाइप बि (हिब)
hair (n)	one of the cylindrical, often colored filaments growing from the skin of a human	रौँ
hairline (n)	the edge of a person's hair, esp. along the top of the forehead	कपाल रेखा
halitosis (n)	a foul odor from the mouth	श्वास गन्हाउने
hallucination (n)	false or distorted perception of objects or events with a compelling sense of reality, usually as a product of mental disorder or as a response to a drug	दृष्टिभ्रम
hand (n) (m)	the end of the human arm below the wrist, consisting of the palm, four fingers, and a thumb	हात
handicapped (adj)	at a disadvantage or suffering from a deficiency, esp. a physical or mental disability that prevents or restricts normal activities	विकलांग

English-Nepali Medical Glossary – H

Term	Definition	Nepali
hangover (n)	unpleasant feeling or sensation following the heavy or over use of alcohol	ह्यांगओभर
Hansen's disease (n)	leprosy; a chronic, infectious disease that causes lumps on the skin	कुष्ठरोग
hardening of the arteries (n)	a condition in which excess cholesterol builds up inside the arteries, causing them to narrow; also referred to as "atherosclerosis"	धमनीहरु कडा हुनु
Hawaiian (n)	a native or resident of Hawaii, especially one of Polynesian ancestry	हवाईको बासिन्दा
hay fever, allergic rhinitis (n)	an acute allergic condition of the eyes and respiratory system, characterized by a running nose, sneezing, and headaches, and often caused by an abnormal sensitivity to certain airborne pollens	पराग ज्वरो, मौसमी ज्वरो
head (n)	the uppermost part of the body, containing the brain, ears, eyes, mouth, and jaw	टाउको
headache (n)	a pain in the head	टाउको दुख्नु
heal (v)	to restore to health or soundness; to cure	निको हुनु
health (n)	the overall condition of a person at any given time	स्वास्थ्य
health care (n)	the prevention, treatment, and management of illness and the preservation of mental and physical well-being through the services offered by the medical and health professions	स्वास्थ्य सेवा

English-Nepali Medical Glossary – H

Term	Definition	Nepali
Health Care Agency (n)	a local administrative entity responsible for providing public and preventive health services to the citizens	स्वास्थ्य सेवा निकाय
Health Care Financing Administration (HCFA) (n)	The federal agency responsible for administering Medicare and overseeing State administration of Medicaid. HCFA is now known as CMS – Center for Medicaid & State Operations	हेल्थ केयर फाइनान्सिङ्ग एडमिनिस्ट्रेसन (एच.सी.एफ.ए.)
health care provider (n)	a person or institution (i.e. doctor, nurse, hospital, insurance company, health maintenance organization) that provides health care services to people	स्वास्थ्य सेवा प्रदायक
health care services (n)	services provided with the purpose of taking care of the health of individuals	स्वास्थ्य सेवाहरु
Health Consumer Action Center (HCAC) (n)	an advocy group working to protect the rights of consumers	हेल्थ कन्जुमर एक्सन सेन्टर (एच.सी.ए.सी.)
health educator (n)	a practitioner who is professionally prepared in the field of health education, who demonstrates competence in both theory and practice, and who accepts responsibility to advance the aims of the health education profession	स्वास्थ्य शिक्षक
Health Insuring Organization (HIO) (n)	A local, public agency which receives all Medicaid funding that would be spent on eligibles in its area: arranges for the provision of all necessary medical services; and pays providers for those services	स्वास्थ्य वीमा संगठन (एच.आई.ओ.)

English-Nepali Medical Glossary – H

Term	Definition	Nepali
Health Maintenance Organization (HMO) (n)	an entity that provides, offers or arranges for coverage of designated health services needed by plan members for a fixed, prepaid premium. There are four basis models of HMOs: staff model, group model, network model and individual practice association	स्वास्थ्य रेखदेख संगठन (एच.एम.ओ.)
health network (n)	a group of health care professionals working with a hospital to provide services to patients under a contract with a health plan	स्वास्थ्य सन्जाल
Healthy Families Program (HFP) (n)	a state and federal funded health coverage program for children under the age of 19	हेल्थी फ्यामेलीज प्रोग्राम (एच.एफ.पी.)
hear (v)	to perceive by the ear; to listen	सुन्नु
hearing aid (n)	an instrument placed in the ear to increase the sound level for a person who hears poorly	सुन्न मद्दत गर्ने साधन
hearing loss (n)	a condition of not being able to hear or sense sound; reduction in the ability to hear	कान नसुन्नु
heart (n)	the hollow, muscular organ that pumps blood from veins to arteries and provides blood to the entire body	मुटु
heart attack (n)	myocardial infarction or death of an area of heart muscle from lack of blood reaching the muscle, often due to coronary artery disease	हृदयघात
heart defects (n)	any of numerous conditions where the heart does not function properly	मुटुका खराबीहरु

Term	Definition	Nepali
heart disease (n)	occurs when blood vessels supplying blood to the heart muscle (the coronary arteries) are narrowed or blocked; the narrowing or blockage is most often caused by buildup of fat (cholesterol) and calcium inside the heart arteries	मुटुको रोग
heart failure (n)	the inability of the heart to pump blood	हृदयघात
heart murmur (n)	noise, heard usually with a stethoscope, that is caused by turbulent blood flow in the heart; may be normal or associated with heart or valvular disease	मुटुमा रगत बगेको आवाज
heart rate (n)	the number of heart beats per unit of time, usually per minute	मुटुको धड्कनको गति
heart trouble (n)	any difficulty, distress, disease, malfunction, etc., of the heart	मुटुको समस्या
heart valve (n)	one of several openings in the heart that controls the flow of blood into other chambers or areas of the heart	मुटुको भल्भ
heartbeat (n)	a single contraction of the heart	धड्कन
heartburn (n)	a burning sensation caused by stomach acids backing up into the lower esophagus (the tube that leads from the mouth to the stomach); the acids produce a burning sensation and discomfort between the ribs just below the breast bone	मुटुपोल्नु
heat (n)	a sensation of feeling hot; the condition of being hot	ताप
heat exhaustion (n)	a reaction to excessive heat, marked by weakness and collapse resulting from a lack of water	धपेडी हुनु

English-Nepali Medical Glossary – H

Term	Definition	Nepali
heat stroke (n)	a severe illness caused by exposure to excessively high temperatures and characterized by severe headache, high fever, dry hot skin, and, in serious cases, collapse and coma	लू लाग्नु
heel (n)	the rounded end portion of the foot under and behind the ankle	कुर्कुच्चा
height (n)	a measurement of how tall someone is; stature, esp. of the human body	उचाई
hematological (adj)	relating to hematology, the branch of medical science which treats diseases of the blood and blood-forming tissues	रगत विज्ञान सम्बन्धी
hematologist (n)	a person who specializes in the science encompassing the generation, anatomy, physiology, pathology, and therapeutics of blood	रगत विज्ञ
hematology (n)	the scientific study of the generation, anatomy, physiology, pathology, and therapeutics of blood	रगत विज्ञान
hematoma (n)	a localized collection of blood, usually clotted, in an organ, space, or tissue, due to a break in the wall of a blood vessel	रगत जमेको, निलडाम
hemiplegia (n)	paralysis of one side of the body, sometimes caused by a stroke	एकतर्फको पक्षघात
hemodialysis (n)	a filtration process to remove toxic substances from the blood in cases of kidney disorders	हेमोडायलाइसिस
hemoglobin (n)	a protein found in red blood cells that carries oxygen	हेमोग्लोबिन
hemophilia (n)	a hereditary condition characterized by the inability to stop bleeding	हेमोफिलिया

English-Nepali Medical Glossary – H

Term	Definition	Nepali
hemopoietic system (n)	the system of tissues and organs, including bone marrow, that are responsible for the production and development of blood cells	रक्तनिर्माण प्रणाली
hemorrhage (n)	escape of blood from the vessels; bleeding	रक्तश्राव
hemorrhoids (n)	an itching or painful mass of swollen veins at the anus	पाइल्स
hepatic (adj)	of, or pertaining to the liver	कलेजोको
hepatitis (n)	inflammation of the liver	कलेजोको सुजन
Hepatitis A (n)	inflammation of the liver caused by the hepatitis A virus (HAV), which is usually transmitted by food or drink that has been handled by an infected person whose hygiene is poor; symptoms include nausea, fever, and jaundice (yellowing of the skin and/or eyes)	हेपाटाइटिस ए
Hepatitis B (n)	inflammation of the liver due to the hepatitis B virus (HBV) once thought to be passed only through blood products; it is now known that hepatitis B can also be transmitted via needle sticks, body piercing, and tattooing using unsterilized instruments, the dialysis process, sexual and even less intimate close contact, and childbirth; symptoms include fatigue, jaundice, nausea, vomiting, dark urine, and light stools	हेपाटाइटिस बी

English-Nepali Medical Glossary – H

Term	Definition	Nepali
herb (n)	a plant that has a fleshy stem, as distinguished from the woody tissue of shrubs and trees, and that generally dies back at the end of each growing season; any of various plants that smell, esp. in medicine	जडीबुटी
herbalist (n)	one versed in herbal lore and, in regard to therapy, an herb doctor	बैध्य
hereditary (n)	derived or transmitted from an ancestor or parent, esp. referring to a disorder or disease	वंशानुगत
heredity (n)	genetic transmission of a particular quality or trait from parent to offspring	आनुवंशिकता
hermetic (adj)	completely sealed, esp. against the escape or entry of air	वायुरोधी
hernia (n)	protrusion of a loop or knuckle of an organ or tissue through an abnormal opening	हर्निया
herniated disk (n)	the dislocation of cartilage found between two vertebrae in the spinal cord or back bone	मेरुदण्डको हर्निया
herpes (n)	an inflammatory skin disease caused by the herpes virus, characterized by the eruption of blisters on the skin	हर्पिस
herpes sore, cold sore, fever blister (n)	a painful eruption or blister on the skin caused by a herpes infection	दाद, फोका, खटिरा
hiccup (n)	a spasm of the diaphragm resulting in a sudden inhalation that is stopped by a rapid closing of the airway to the lungs	बाडुली
high blood pressure (n)	an increased or abnormally high level of pressure in the arteries	उच्च रक्तचाप

English-Nepali Medical Glossary – H

Term	Definition	Nepali
hip (n)	the body part that projects sideways from the pelvis or pelvic region between the waist to the thigh	कमर, नितम्ब
Hispanics/Latinos (n)	a person of Latin-American origin living in the U.S.	ल्याटिन अमेरिकी
histology (n)	the study of the physical structure of tissue	तन्तुशास्त्र
history (medical) (n) (m)	a narrative of events; story; a chronological record of events, often including an explanation of or commentary on those events, esp. a record of a patient's medical background	इतिहास (चिकित्सा)
HIV (n)	acronym for the Human Immunodeficiency Virus, the cause of AIDS (acquired immunodeficiency syndrome)	एच.आई.भी
hives (n)	a skin condition characterized by intensely itching welts and caused by allergic reactions to internal or external agents	चिलाउने खटिरा
hoarse (adj)	having a husky and grating voice	धोद्रो
hobby (n)	a pastime	अभिरुचि
hold on (v)	to grasp or squeeze an object	समात्नु
hold your breath (v)	to refrain from expelling air from the lungs for a period of time	सास रोक्नु
holter monitor (n)	small portable ECG device for long-term recording of electrical activity of the heart; may detect fleeting changes that might otherwise go unnoticed	होल्टर मनिटर
Home Delivery Meals (HDM) (n)	meals delivered to ones home due to infirmity or illness	होम डेलिभरी मिल्स (एच.डी.एम.)

English-Nepali Medical Glossary – H

Term	Definition	Nepali
home maker chores (n)	household services, including household cleaning, laundry, shopping, food preparation, and household maintenance	घरायसी सेवाहरु
hormone (n)	a chemical substance produced in the body that controls and regulates the activity of certain cells or organs	हर्मोन
hormone replacement therapy (n)	a combination therapy of estrogen plus progesterone, used to treat menopause	हर्मोन रिप्लेसमेंट थेरापी
hormone therapy (n)	a process of treating a disease with medication containing specific hormones	हर्मोन थेरापी
hospice (n)	an establishment or a program that provides for the physical and emotional needs of terminally ill patients	धर्मशाला
hospital (n)	an institution that provides medical or surgical care and treatment for the sick and the injured	अस्पताल
hospitalization (n)	confinement of a patient in a hospital, or the period of such confinement	अस्पतालमा भर्ना गर्नु
hot flashes (n)	a passing symptom of menopause that involves the sensation of heat all over the body	शरीर पोल्ने
hot pack (n)	a sac or pouch that becomes warm from an internal chemical reaction and is placed on the skin to promote blood circulation	तातो पोको
hot water bottle (n)	a rubber container filled with hot water used to warm the bed or parts of the body	तातो बोतल
humerus (n)	the long bone of the upper arm	पाखुराको हड्डी

English-Nepali Medical Glossary – H

Term	Definition	Nepali
hurt (v)	to cause physical damage or pain; to injure	चोट लगाउनु
hydration (n)	condition of being combined with water	जलयोजन
hydrocephalus (n)	a condition in which an abnormal accumulation of fluid in the brain causes enlargement of the skull and compression of the brain	टाउकोमा पानी भरिनु
hydrogen peroxide (n)	a colorless, heavy, liquid used principally to clean wounds and medical equipment	हाइड्रोजन पेरोक्साइड
hygiene (n)	prevention of disease through cleanliness	स्वच्छता
hymen (n)	a fold of tissue partly or completely blocking the opening of the vagina; normal, not pathologic	योनिद्वारको झिल्ली
hyperactivity (n)	the state of being excessively active, moving more than normal	सक्रियता
hyperglycemia (n)	a condition of a high level of sugar in the blood; see related words including sugar, glucose, and carbohydrate	हाइपरग्लाइसेमिया
hyperopia (n)	a condition in which the eye does not focus properly on objects at close range without the assistance of glasses; farsightedness	हाइपरओपिया
hypertension (n)	continuously high blood pressure	उच्च रक्तचाप
hyperthermia (n)	abnormally high body temperature, especially that induced for therapeutic purposes	उच्चताप, गर्मी
hyperthyroidism (n)	excessive functional activity of the thyroid gland; overproduction of thyroid hormone; opposite of hypothyroidism	हाइपरथाइरोइडीजम

English-Nepali Medical Glossary – H

Term	Definition	Nepali
hyperventilation (n)	a state in which there is an increased amount of air entering the lungs	उच्च श्वासप्रश्वास दर
hypnosis (n)	an induced sleeplike condition in which an individual is extremely responsive to suggestions made by the person causing this condition	सम्मोहन
hypnotize (v)	to put in a state of hypnosis	सम्मोहित गर्नु
hypochondriasis (n)	the continued belief that one is or is likely to become ill, often involving experiences of real pain, when illness is neither present nor likely	हाइपोथकोंड्रीएसिस्
hypodermic (adj)	applied or administered beneath the skin	हाइपोडरमिक, छालामुनि
hypoglycemia (n)	a low level of sugar in the blood; see related words including sugar, glucose, and carbohydrate	हईपोग्लाइसेमिया
hypothermia (n)	a low body temperature, as that due to exposure in cold weather or induced as a means of decreasing metabolism as used in various surgical procedures	जाडो लाग्नु
hypothyroidism (n)	reduction of thyroid activity, esp. the release of hormones	हाइपोथाइरोइडीजम
hysterectomy (n)	operation of removing the uterus, and sometimes, ovaries, performed either through the abdominal wall or through the vagina	गर्भाशय हटाउनु

English-Nepali Medical Glossary – I

Term	Definition	Nepali
iatrogenic (adj)	resulting from the activity of physicians	आइट्रोजेनिक
ICD-9 Codes/Coding System (n)	International Classification of Diseases (ICD-9) is a universally accpeted standard coding system utilized by healthcare providers to assist in preparing bills and adjudicating claims payment	आई.सी.डी.-९ कोड/कोडीङ प्रणाली
ice pack (n)	a cold instrument used to cool the body and reduce the blood supply to an area	आइस प्याक
idiosyncrasy (n)	an abnormal sensitivity to some drug, protein, or other agent	सनक, स्वभाव
ileum (n)	the last portion of the small intestine	सानो आन्द्राको अन्तिम भाग
immaturity (n)	state or quality of being not fully developed	अपरिपक्वता
immobilization (n)	act of rendering not movable, as by a cast or splint	स्थिरीकरण
immune (adj)	protected against infectious disease	मुक्त, सुरक्षित
immune system (n)	the activity, organs, glands, and structures in the body responsible for providing protection against disease	प्रतिरक्षा प्रणाली
immunity (n)	protection against infectious disease	प्रतिरक्षा
immunization (n)	the process of making someone immune to a disease, usually by injection of some substance	खोप कार्य
immunization schedule (n)	a calendar of recommended shots	खोप तालिका
immunize (v)	to render immune by injection (or oral medication)	खोप लगाउनु

English-Nepali Medical Glossary – I

Term	Definition	Nepali
immunology (n)	the medical study of the immune system and how it protects the body against infectious disease	इम्युनोलोजी
impaired (adj)	reduced in strength, value, quantity, or quality	खराब
impaired vision (n)	the inability to see clearly	दृष्टिको खराबी
impetigo (n)	a skin infection caused by a specific bacteria characterized by blisters that erupt and form yellow crusts	चर्मरोग
implant (n) (m)	something implanted, esp. surgically implanted tissue	प्रत्यारोपण गरिएको बस्तु
implant (v) (m)	to insert or embed surgically	प्रत्यारोपण
implantation (n)	insertion or grafting into the body of biological, living, inert, or radioactive material	प्रत्यारोपण कार्य
implication (n)	a possible effect of an action	आशय
impotence (n)	the condition of not being able to perform sexual intercourse, inability to get or maintain an erect penis; lacking physical strength or vigor	नपुंसकता
impregnation (n)	the act of rendering pregnant	गर्भवती बनाउने काम
in situ (adj/adv)	in the original place; may refer to the origin of a cancerous tumor	यथास्थानमा
in vitro (adv)	within a glass; observable in a test tube; in an artificial environment	इन भिट्रो
inactive (adj)	not active; being out of use	निष्क्रिय
incarceration (n) (m)	abnormal retention or confinement of a body part	रोक, बन्दी
incision (n)	a surgical cut into soft tissue; the act of cutting into or marking with a sharp instrument	चिरा

English-Nepali Medical Glossary – I

Term	Definition	Nepali
incisor (n)	a tooth adapted for cutting, located at the front of the mouth	टोक्ने दाँत
incompetence (n)	physical or mental inadequacy or insufficiency	असक्षमता
incontinence (n)	inability to control excretory functions, as defecation or urination	अनियंत्रण
incubation (n)	a time of growth	सङ्क्रमण
incubation period (n)	the length of time required for symptoms to be visible after entrance of a disease into the body	सङ्क्रमण काल
incubator (n)	a cabinet in which a uniform temperature can be maintained, used in growing bacteria, or in keeping small babies warm	इनक्यूबेटर
index finger (n)	the finger next to the thumb	चोर औला
indication (n)	a sign or circumstance which points to or shows the cause, pathology, issue, or an attack of a disease	संकेत
indigestion (n)	inability to eat or digest something, esp. food; discomfort or illness resulting from indigestion	अपच
induce (v)	to cause something to happen, esp. by the administration of medication	गराउनु
induced abortion (n)	a procedure or drug that causes an abortion	गर्भपात गराउनु
induced labor (n)	the act or process of causing a woman to begin the birthing of a child through medication or other medical procedure	प्रसब गराउनु
induced vomiting (n)	a procedure or drug that causes vomiting	बान्ता गराउनु

English-Nepali Medical Glossary – I

Term	Definition	Nepali
infantile (adj)	pertaining to an infant or to infancy	शिशुको जस्तो
infantile paralysis (n)	poliomyelitis; an infectious viral disease occurring mainly in children and in its acute form attacking the central nervous system and producing paralysis	पोलियो
infarct (n)	the death of tissue caused by a lack of blood to the tissue	इन्फार्क्ट
infect (v)	to have microorganisms enter the body and produce harmful toxins	संक्रमित पार्नु
infected (adj)	of, or pertaining to a person who has a disease	संक्रमित
infection (n)	the invasion and multiplication of microorganisms in body tissues	सङ्क्रमण
infectious disease (n)	germs that invade the body and create an infection that can spread from person to person	सङ्क्रामक रोग
infertility (n)	the inability to reproduce	बाँझोपन
infiltration (n) (m)	the accumulation of a substance in a tissue or cell	घुसपैठ
inflammation (n)	localized heat, redness, swelling, and pain as a result of irritation, injury, or infection	सुजन
influenza (n)	acute viral infection involving the respiratory tract	इन्फ्लुएन्जा
informed consent (n)	the process of informing, educating, or telling a patient about a medical treatment (esp. the risks of undergoing the treatment), ascertaining the patient's understanding of this information, and obtaining the written permission for the treatment from the patient	सुचित सहमति
infuse (v)	to pour a liquid into something	खन्याउनु

English-Nepali Medical Glossary – I

Term	Definition	Nepali
infusion (n)	therapeutic introduction of a fluid other than blood, as saline solution, into a vein	प्रक्षेपण
ingestion (n)	the act of taking food, medicine, etc., into the body, by mouth	खुवाई
ingrown toenail (n)	a toenail that has grown into the skin causing inflammation	गढेको नङ
inguinal (adj)	of, or relating to, or located between the legs, or in the crease between the legs and the trunk	दूई खुट्टा बिचको
inhalation (n)	drawing of air or other substances into the lungs	सास तान्ने काम
inhale (v)	to draw in by breathing	सास लिनु
inhaler (n)	a device that produces a vapor to ease breathing or to medicate by inspiration	इन्हेलर
injection (n)	forcing a liquid into a part, as into the skin, a vein, or an organ, by a needle	सूई
injure (v)	to cause harm to; to hurt	चोट लगाउनु
injured (adj)	pertaining to someone who sustained an injury	घाइते
injury (n)	damage of or to a person, property, or thing	चोट
inner ear (n)	the portion of the ear that senses position for balance	भित्रि कान
inoculate (v)	to inject a substance into a person to produce an immunity against a disease	खोप लगाउनु
inorganic (adj)	not of organic origin; not of living matter	अजैबिक
inpatient (n)	a patient staying in a hospital for treatment	अन्तरंग बिरामी
insane (adj)	exhibiting, or afflicted with insanity	पागल
insanity (n)	persistent mental disorder	पागलपन

English-Nepali Medical Glossary – I

Term	Definition	Nepali
insect bite (n)	the mark left on the skin from the bite of an insect	किराको टोकाई
insecticide (n)	a substance, chemical, or agent that kills insects	किटनाशक
insert (v)	to introduce into the body; to place inside	घुसार्नु
insertion (n)	place of attachment, as of a muscle to the bone which it moves	टाँसिएको ठाउँ
insidious (adj)	of, or pertaining to a disease that develops without symptoms	लक्षण रहित
insomnia (n)	inability to sleep; abnormal wakefulness	अनिद्रा
inspiration (n)	act of drawing air into the lungs	श्वास लिने काम
instability (n)	quality or state of being unstable or without balance	अस्थिरता
instep (n)	the arched portion of the foot	पैतालाको भित्रि भाग
insulin (n)	a hormone that controls the level of sugar in the blood	इन्सुलिन
insulin reaction or shock (n)	low level of sugar in the blood caused by excessive insulin	इन्सुलिनको प्रतिक्रिया वा आघात
insult (n)	injury or trauma; attack, harmful action	आक्रमण
insurance (n)	coverage by a contract binding a party to pay for loss of another party, esp. insurance that covers medical expenses	बीमा
insurance company (n)	a business that sells insurance	बीमा कम्पनी
intact (adj)	the condition of having something functional, complete, and living; having no relevant component removed or destroyed	यथावत, जस्ताको तस्तै
intensive care (n)	special medical equipment and services provided for seriously ill patients; a hospital unit that specializes in intensive care	सघन उपचार

English-Nepali Medical Glossary – I

Term	Definition	Nepali
interaction (n)	quality, state, or process of two or more things acting on each other	अन्तरक्रिया
intercourse (n)	1. dealings or communications between persons or groups; 2. sexual intercourse	समागम
intermediary (adj)	performed or occurring in a middle stage; neither early or late; intermediate	मध्यस्थ
intermittent (adj)	occurring at separated intervals; having periods of lacking activity	रोकिंदै
internal (adj)	situated or occurring within or on the inside	आन्तरिक
internal bleeding (n)	the abnormal loss of blood into a cavity inside the body	आन्तरिक रक्तश्राव
internal medicine (n)	a medical specialty dedicated to the prevention, diagnosis, and treatment of diseases of adults	रोकथाम चिकित्सा
internist (n)	a physician who specializes in internal medicine, the medical study and treatment of non-surgical diseases in adults	रोकथाम चिकित्सा विशेषज्ञ
interpretation (n)	the act, process, or result of interpreting from one language to another in order to convey the meaning of a statement	व्याख्या
interpreter (n)	one who translates orally from one language into another	दोभाषे
intervention (n)	act or fact of interfering so as to modify	हस्तक्षेप
intestinal (adj)	referring to the intestines	आन्द्राको
intestines (n)	the portion of the digestive system extending from the stomach to the anus	आन्द्राहरु
intoxicated (adj)	having excess of a toxin, esp. excess alcohol	नसा लागेको
intramuscular (adj)	within or inside muscle tissue	मांसपेशीमा

English-Nepali Medical Glossary – I

Term	Definition	Nepali
intraocular (adj)	within the eye	आँखामा
intrauterine device (n)	an object that is placed within the uterus to prevent pregnancy	पाठेघरमा राखिने उपकरण
intravenous (adj)	within a vein or veins	शिरामा, नसामा
intravenous pyelography (n)	an examination of the kidneys by injecting a liquid visible using x-rays	इन्ट्राभेनस पाएलोग्राफि
intravenous transfusion (n)	the direct injection of whole blood, plasma, or another solution into the blood stream	इन्ट्राभेनस ट्रान्सफ्युजन
intubation (n)	insertion of a tube into a body canal or hollow organ, as into the trachea or stomach	नली घुसार्ने काम
invasive (adj)	involving puncture or incision of the skin or insertion of an instrument or foreign material into the body	चोटपटक युक्त
inverted nipples (n)	nipples that are turned inward	गढेको स्तनको मुन्टो
iodine (n)	a grayish-black, corrosive, poisonous element used to clean the skin	आयोडिन
iris (n)	the colored, round, membrane of the eye, situated between the cornea and lens	आँखाको नानी
iritis (n)	inflammation of the iris	आँखाको नानी सुन्निने
iron supplements (n)	an oral medication used to supply the body with additional iron	फलाम तत्वको खुराक
irregular (adj)	not normal; not straight or uniform; having an uneven rate	अनियमत
irrigation (n)	washing by a stream of water or other fluid	सिँचाई
irritants (n)	something that causes inflammation, soreness, or irritation of a bodily organ or part	सन्तापक, दाहक

English-Nepali Medical Glossary – I

Term	Definition	Nepali
irritation (n)	state of over-excitation and extreme sensitivity	झर्को
ischemia (n)	deficiency of blood in a part, due to functional constriction or actual obstruction of a blood vessel	इस्केमिया
itch (n)	a skin sensation causing a desire to scratch	कन्याउने इच्छा
itch (v)	to feel, have or produce an itch	कन्याउनु

English-Nepali Medical Glossary – J

Term	Definition	Nepali
jaundice (n)	yellow discoloration of skin, tissues, and body fluids caused by the deposition of bile pigments arising from a variety of conditions that affect the liver	जन्डिस, कमलपित्त
jaw (n)	the bone holding the lower teeth	बंगारा च्यापु
jejunum (n)	the middle portion of the small intestine which extends from the duodenum to the ileum	सानो आन्द्राको बिचको भाग
jelly (n)	a soft, semi-solid substance used as lubrication and sometimes containing medication or other chemicals, such as spermicidal jelly	थलथले, जेल्ली
joint (n)	a point of connection between more or less movable parts, between bones, or between segments in the bone	जोर्नि
joint socket (n)	the hollow part of a joint that receives the end of a bone	जोर्नीको प्वाल

English-Nepali Medical Glossary – K

Term	Definition	Nepali
keratitis (n)	inflammation of the cornea causing poor vision and pain	आँखाको सुजन
kidney (n)	either of a pair of structures in the back region of the abdominal cavity, functioning to maintain proper water balance, regulate acid-base concentration, and excrete wastes as urine	मृगौला
kidney failure (n)	loss of function of one or both kidneys, usually caused by disease or infection	मृगौलाले काम नगर्नु
kidney stone (n)	a small hard mass that has formed in the kidney and may block the ureter	मृगौलाको पत्थरी
kilogram (n)	the fundamental unit of mass in the International System, equaling 2.2 pounds	किलोग्राम
knee (n)	the joint or region of the human leg that is between the thigh and calf	घुँडा
kneecap (n)	patella; a bone that rests on the knee	घुँडाको पांग्रा
knuckle (n)	a joint in the finger, esp. the joint where the finger connects to the hand	औंलाको जोर्नि
kyphosis (n)	hunchback; humpback; excessive curve in the back and spine	कुप्रो

English-Nepali Medical Glossary – L

Term	Definition	Nepali
labor (n) (m)	the physical efforts of childbirth	प्रसव
labor and delivery (n)	1. an obstetrical unit, usually associated with prepartum (labor) rooms, a delivery unit (rooms) where child birth occurs and post partum areas where a new mother recovers and begins to care for her child; 2. a term that refers to the physiology of child bearing as in a lecture entitled, "The physiology of normal labor and delivery," or to the active process of bearing a child	प्रसव र जन्म
labor pains (n)	pain associated with childbirth	प्रसव पिडा
laboratory (n)	a room or building equipped for scientific experiment, research, or the evaluation of blood specimens	प्रयोगशाला
laboratory technician (n)	a person trained to work and conduct experiments in a laboratory	प्रयोगशाला प्राविधिक
laboratory test (n)	any of various tests conducted in a laboratory to assist in the diagnosis of a disease	प्रयोगशाला परिक्षण
labyrinth (n)	the complex section of passages in the inner ear that senses sound and maintains balance	कान भित्रको भाग
laceration (n)	a torn, ragged, mangled wound	कोतारिएको घाऊ
lacrimal gland (n)	a gland near the eye that secretes tears	अश्रु ग्रंथि
lactation (n)	the act of secreting milk	दुध निकाल्नु
lactose intolerance (n)	the inability of the body to digest a specific sugar, lactose; this condition is associated with an upset stomach, diarrhea, and stomach pains	ल्याक्टोज इन्टोलरेंस

English-Nepali Medical Glossary – L

Term	Definition	Nepali
laparoscope (n)	an instrument used to view inside the abdominal cavity	लेपारोस्कोप
laparoscopic (adj)	of, or pertaining to a medical procedure of visually examining the abdominal cavity with a slender camera	लेपारोस्कोपको
large intestine (n)	the section of the digestive system between the small intestine and anus, consisting of the cecum, colon, rectum, and anal canal	ठुलो आन्द्रा
laryngitis (n)	inflammation of the larynx, a condition causing dryness and soreness of the throat, hoarseness, and cough	गलाको सुजन
laryngoscope (n)	a tubular instrument or apparatus used to observe the interior of the larynx	ल्यारिन्गोस्कोप
larynx (n)	the upper part of the respiratory tract containing the vocal cords	गला
laser surgery, laser photo-coagulation (n)	a surgical procedure using a small laser to destroy tissue or make incisions	लेजर शल्यक्रिया
latent period (n)	seemingly inactive period, as that between exposure of tissue to an injurious agent and the manifestation of response, or that between a stimulation and the response to the stimulus	निष्क्रिय अवधि
laxative (n)	agent that acts to promote release of feces	रेचक, दिशा लगाउने
lay hands on (v)	the act of resting a person's hand in a particular position or location; a belief that a person has the power to heal through touch	हात राख्नु
lead poisoning (n)	the pathological effects of ingesting or absorbing lead	सिसाको बिषाक्तता

English-Nepali Medical Glossary – L

Term	Definition	Nepali
leads (n) (m)	a wire that connects a monitoring device to a patient	तारहरु
leg (n)	a limb or appendage used for movement or support	खुट्टा
lens (n) (m)	a carefully ground and molded piece of glass, plastic, or other transparent material used for changing the size or shape of an image	लेन्स
lens (n) (m)	a transparent part of the eye between the iris and the vitreous used to direct light onto the retina	आँखाको लेन्स
leprosy (n)	an infectious disease usually occurring in the tropics, which can range from being non-contagious to contagious, causing deterioration of the skin; Hansen's disease	कुष्ठरोग
lesion (n)	a mark on the skin, or abnormal growth (tumor)	घाउ, दाग
lethal (adj)	deadly; fatal	घातक
lethargy (n)	1. abnormal drowsiness or stupor; 2. a condition of indifference	अल्छीपन
leukemia (n)	an acute or chronic disease that involves the blood-forming organs; a form of cancer	रगतको क्यान्सर
libido (n)	sexual desire	यौन चाहना
lice (n)	any of numerous small, flatbodied, wingless, biting or sucking insects, usually found in hair	जुम्रा

Term	Definition	Nepali
licensed practical nurse (n)	a graduate of a school of practical nursing who has passed the practical nursing state board examination and is licensed to administer care, usually working under direction of a licensed physician or registered nurse	लाइसन्स प्राप्त नर्स
life support (n)	hospital equipment that maintains the life of a patient who might not be able to survive independently	प्राण बचाइराख्ने यन्त्र
lifestyle (n)	a way of life or style of living that reflects the attitudes and values of an individual or group	जीवन शैली
ligament (n)	a band of fibrous tissue that connects bones or cartilage, serving to support and strengthen joints	अस्थीबन्धन
limbs (n)	one of the jointed appendages of the human, extending from the trunk	हातखुट्टा
limit (n)	a prescribed maximum or minimum amount, quantity, or number	सीमा
limp (v)	to walk lamely, esp. with irregularity, as in favoring one leg	लडखडाउनु
lip (n)	either of two fleshy, muscular folds that together surround the opening of the mouth	ओठ
liquids (n)	fluids	तरल पदार्थहरु
little finger (n)	the smallest finger on the hand and most distant from the thumb	हातको कान्छीऔंला
little toe (n)	the smallest toe on the foot and most distant from the big toe	खुट्टाको कान्छीऔंला

English-Nepali Medical Glossary – L

Term	Definition	Nepali
liver (n)	a large gland that secretes bile, helps in blood formation, and is involved in the metabolism of sugars, fats, proteins, minerals, and vitamins	कलेजो
liver cancer (n)	a tumor in which the cancer starts during adulthood in cells in the liver; also called hepatocellular carcinoma	कलेजोको क्यान्सर
living will (n)	a legal document that outlines actions that should be taken if the author is seriously ill and can no longer express wishes regarding his or her death	इच्छापत्र
loading dose (n)	a quantity higher than the average or maintenance dose, for starting a treatment	सुरुको मात्र
lobe (n)	more or less well-defined portion of any organ, especially of the brain, lungs, glands, and ear lobe	खण्ड, भाग
local (adj)	restricted to one spot or part	स्थानीय
local anesthesia (n)	anesthetic which causes loss of feeling only on and around the point where it is applied or injected	स्थानीय संज्ञाहरण
long term care facility (n)	a health care facility that serves patients with medical conditions requiring nursing and/or medical care on an extended basis	दीर्घकालीन रेखदेख सुबिधा
lose consciousness (v)	to become unconscious, without awareness, and not capable of voluntary movement	होश गुमाउनु
lose weight (v)	to lower body weight through exercise, dieting, or disease	तौल घटाउनु

English-Nepali Medical Glossary – L

Term	Definition	Nepali
lotion (n)	a medicated liquid for external application	लोसन
low voice (n)	a voice that is not loud; silent	मसिनो बोली
lower (adj)	below something or someone; below a particular level	तल्लो
lower back, lumbar (n)	the region of the back behind the stomach and above the waist	तल्लो ढाड
lower jaw (n)	mandible; the movable bone forming the chin and lower portion of the face; it is used in chewing and crushing food	तल्लो बंगारा
lubricant (n)	an oily substance, such as grease, that reduces friction, heat, and wear when applied as a surface coating	स्निग्धकारी
lukewarm (adj)	mildly warm	मनतातो
lumbar (adj)	the lower back between the ribs and the pelvis	ढाडको
lumbar puncture, spinal tap (n)	the removal of fluid from the spine to assist in diagnosing a disease, such as meningitis	ढाडमा सियो घुसार्ने काम
lump (n)	a swelling or small mass	गाँठो
lumpectomy (n)	the removal of a lump	गाँठो हटाउनु
lung (n)	either of two spongy, saclike respiratory organs occupying the chest cavity together with the heart, and functioning to remove carbon dioxide from the blood and provide the body with oxygen	फोक्सो

English-Nepali Medical Glossary – L

Term	Definition	Nepali
lung cancer (n)	cancer of the lung which is not of the small cell carcinoma (oat cell carcinoma) type; this is generally applied to the various types of bronchogenic carcinomas (those arising from the lining of the bronchi) which include adenocarcinoma, squamous cell carcinoma, and large cell undifferentiated carcinoma	फोक्सोको क्यान्सर
lung scan (n)	a procedure in which radiation material is injected into the blood to diagnose diseases of the lungs	फोक्सोको अवलोकन
lymph (n)	a clear, transparent, sometimes faintly yellowish liquid that contains white blood cells and some red blood cells and acts to remove bacteria and certain proteins from tissues	लसीका
lymph glands (n)	lymph nodes; glands found throughout the body that produce a clear, transparent, sometimes faintly yellowish liquid that contains white blood cells and some red blood cells and acts to remove bacteria and certain proteins from tissues; involved in fighting infection	लसीका ग्रन्थीहरु
lymphadenopathy (n)	enlargement of the lymph nodes	लसीका ग्रन्थीहरुको सुजन
lymphatic system (n)	the interconnected system of spaces and vessels between tissues and organs by which lymph is circulated throughout the body	लसीका प्रणाली
lymphoma (n)	a cancerous tumor of lymphoid tissue	लसीका तन्तुको क्यान्सर

English-Nepali Medical Glossary – M

Term	Definition	Nepali
magnetic resonance imaging (n)	MRI: a diagnostic procedure using magnetic fields (rather than x-ray radiation) to create an image of internal soft tissue, such as muscle, brain, and spinal cord	म्याग्नेटिक रिजोनेन्स इमेजिंग
major depression (n)	a state of depression which includes symptoms of lethargy, sleep disturbance, despondency, morbid thoughts, feelings of worthlessness, and sometimes attempted suicide	ठुलो उदासी
malabsorption (n)	impaired intestinal absorption of nutrients	शोषणको खराबी
malaise (n)	a vague feeling of bodily discomfort	अस्वस्थता
malaria (n)	an acute and sometimes chronic disease caused by a microorganism that infects red blood cells, transmitted by the bite of a mosquito	औलो
malignant (adj)	tending to become progressively worse and to result in death, usually referring to cancer or very serious illness	घातक
malnutrition (n)	inadequate nutrition because of defective digestion or inadequate food intake	कुपोषण
malpractice (n)	improper treatment of a patient by a physician, resulting in damage or injury	कुउपचार
mammary (n)	the breast	स्तन
mammography, mammogram (n)	1. the practice of taking an x-ray photograph of the breast; 2. an x-ray photograph of the breast	म्यामोग्राफि, म्यामोग्राम
manage (v)	to handle or direct with a degree of skill; to work upon or try to alter for a purpose	प्रवन्धन गर्नु

English-Nepali Medical Glossary – M

Term	Definition	Nepali
managed care (n)	a comprehensive approach to the provision of health care that combines clinical services and administrative procedures within an integrated, coordinated system to provide timely access to primary care and other necessary services cost effectively	प्रवन्धित हेरचाह
Managed Care Organization (MCO) (n)	a system of affiliated hospitals, physicians, and others using managed care	प्रवन्धित हेरचाह संगठन (एम.सी.ओ.)
Managed Health Care Plan (n)	one or more products that integrate financing and management with the delivery of health care services to an enrolled population	प्रवन्धित स्वास्थ्य सेवा योजना
management (n)	control or oversight of something	प्रबंधन
mandible (n)	lower jaw; the movable bone forming the chin and lower portion of the face; it is used in chewing and crushing food	तल्लो बंगारा
mania (n)	a mental disorder characterized by rapidly changing ideas, exaggerated walking stride, increased energy, physical over-activity, and confusion	पागलपन
manic (adj)	affected with mania	पागलपन सम्बन्धित
mass (n)	a unified body of matter with no specific shape, sometimes referring to a tumor	पिण्ड
massage (n)	the systematic therapeutic friction, stroking, and kneading of the body	मसाज
mastectomy (n)	surgical removal of a breast	स्तन काटेर हटाउनु

English-Nepali Medical Glossary – M

Term	Definition	Nepali
mastitis (n)	inflammation of the mammary gland, or breast	थुनेलो
masturbation (n)	self-excitation of the genital organs, usually to orgasm, by manual contact or means other than sexual intercourse	हस्तमैथुन
maternity ward (n)	a location in a hospital where a woman who is preparing to give birth or just gave birth resides	प्रसूति वार्ड
measles (n)	an acute, contagious viral disease, usually occurring in childhood and characterized by red spots on the skin	दादुरा
measure (v)	to determine the dimensions, quantity, or capacity of something	नाप्नु
Medicaid (Title XIX) (n)	authorized by Title XIX of the Social Security Act, the Medicaid program provides medical benefits for certain low-income persons; the state and federal governments jointly administer the program	मेदिकेड (टाईटल एक्स.आई.एक्स.)
medical (adj)	anything having to do with medicine or with the treatment of diseases	चिकित्सा सम्बन्धी
medical alert bracelet (n)	bracelet used for the purpose of identifying the person's medical condition and emergency contact person	मेडिकल अलर्ट ब्रासलेट
medical assistant (n)	an individual who assists a qualified physician in an office or other clinical setting	चिकित्सा सहयोगी
Medical Director (n)	a physician responsible for clinical decisions in a health plan or health network	चिकित्सा निर्देशक
medical history (n)	the medical background of a patient, including allergies, past injuries, and diseases	चिकित्सा इतिहास

English-Nepali Medical Glossary – M

Term	Definition	Nepali
medical necessity (n)	the determination that an intervention recommended by a treating practitioner is (1) the most appropriate available supply or level of service for the individual in question, considering potential benefits and harms to the individual, and (2) known to be effective in improving health outcomes	चिकित्सा आवश्यकता
medical records (n)	an organized database or file that contains the medical history of one or more patients, contained in a paper chart or on a computer	चिकित्सा अभिलेख
medical student (n)	a person who is training to be a physician	चिकित्सा विध्यार्थी
Medicare (Title XVIII) (n)	Title XVIII of the Social Security Act which provides for medical and health services to persons age 65 and older and certain disabled individuals; covered Medicare services include physician, hospital care, home care, ancillary, and extended care facility services coverage for a defined period of time	मेडीकेयर (टाईटल एक्स.भी.आई.आई.आई.)
medication (n)	substance given for healing or treatment purposes	उपचार
medicinal (adj)	having healing qualities	औषधीय
medicine (n)	the science of diagnosing, treating, or preventing disease and other damage to the body or mind	औषधी
medicine chest (n)	a storage container for medicine or remedies	औषधीको बाकस
meditate (v)	to reflect upon; to ponder	ध्यान गर्नु

English-Nepali Medical Glossary – M

Term	Definition	Nepali
meditation (n)	the act or process of meditating	ध्यान
melanoma (n)	a tumor of the skin	छालाको क्यान्सर
melena (n)	the passage of dark (often black) stools stained with blood pigments or with altered blood	रगतयुक्त दिसा
member (n)	a person who belongs to an HMO or other health care provider organization; used interchangeably with enrollee and beneficiary	सदस्य
membrane (n)	thin layer of tissue that covers a surface, lines a cavity or divides a space or organ	झिल्ली
memory (n)	the collection of thoughts or images of past events, experiences, knowledge, ideas, and feelings	स्मरण
menarche (n)	establishment or beginning of menstrual function in a girl or young woman	रजोदर्शन
menopause (n)	the end of menstruation in the human female, usually in mid life	रजोनिवृत्ति
menses (n)	blood and dead cell debris that is discharged from the uterus through the vagina by adult women at approximately monthly intervals between puberty and menopause	महिनावारी
menstrual (adj)	of, or pertaining to menstruation	महिनावारीको
menstrual period (n)	the period of time one experiences menstruation each month	महिनावारीको अवधि
menstruation (n)	the cyclic, physiologic discharge through the vagina of blood and dead cells from the non-pregnant uterus	महिनावारी

English-Nepali Medical Glossary – M

Term	Definition	Nepali
mental (adj)	of, or pertaining to the mind; psychic	मानसिक
mental health (n)	a section of the medical profession that specializes in the study and treatment of diseases and disorders related to the mind	मानसिक स्वास्थ्य
mental health professional (n)	a person whose work is related to mental health care	मानसिक स्वास्थ्यकर्मी
mental hospital (n)	a hospital that specializes in treating the mentally ill	मानसिक अस्पताल
mental illness (n)	any disorder of the mind or psyche	मानसिक रोग
mental retardation (n)	mental deficiency; slowed or delayed mental response or activity	सुस्तमनस्थिति
mesentery (n)	a membranous fold attaching various organs to the body wall	अन्त्रपेशी
metabolism (n)	the complex of physical and chemical processes involved in the maintenance of life	अन्तरदहन
metastasize (v)	to transmit a disease from an original site to one or more sites elsewhere in the body, usually referring to cancer	फैलनु
metastatic (adj)	of, or pertaining to the transmission of a disease (usually cancer) from an original site to one or more sites elsewhere in the body	फैलने खालको
microorganism (n)	a very small organism, not visible by the human eye without mechanical or electronic magnification	सुक्ष्मजीव
microscope (n)	an instrument that uses a combination of lenses to enlarge an image of an object so that it can be seen with the eye	सुक्ष्मदर्शक यन्त्र

English-Nepali Medical Glossary – M

Term	Definition	Nepali
middle ear (n)	the middle section of the ear or tympanic cavity involved in hearing; contains the malleus, incus, and stapes	मध्य कान
middle finger (n)	the second finger from the thumb	माझिऔंला
midwife (n)	a person who assists a pregnant woman in childbirth	सुडेनी
migraine (n)	severe, recurrent headache, usually affecting only one side of the head, characterized by sharp pain and often accompanied by nausea	माइग्रेन, अर्धकपाल
mineral (n)	any of various inorganic elements, that are not from an animal or plant, which may be required to live and function properly	खनिज
mineral supplements (n)	oral medication used to make up for a deficiency in one or more minerals in the body	खनिजको खुराक
miscarriage (n)	a spontaneous, unplanned expulsion of a fetus from the uterus	गर्भपात
misery (n)	a condition or feeling of unhappiness, suffering, or discomfort	दुःख
mobility (n)	1. the extent of one's movement; 2. ability to be moved, or to move freely	गतिशीलता
moderation (n)	within reasonable limits, not excessive or extreme	संयम
modify (v)	to change somewhat the form or qualities of; to alter partially	संशोधन गर्नु
moist heat (n)	heat and moisture applied to the skin	ओसिलो तातो
moisture (n)	liquid on a surface, giving it a damp feeling or sensation	ओस

English-Nepali Medical Glossary – M

Term	Definition	Nepali
molar (n)	a tooth with a surface for grinding food, located in the back of the mouth	बंगारा
mold (n) (m)	a frame or mold around or on which something is formed or shaped	साँचो
mold (n) (m)	any of various fungous growths	ढुसी
mole, blemish (n)	a small congenital growth on the skin, usually slightly raised and dark, and sometimes hairy	कोठी
monitor (n) (m)	an instrument used to keep track of an activity, esp. to record the activity of the lungs, brain, or heart	मनिटर
mononucleosis (n)	a temporary illness associated with fatigue and abnormal white blood cells in the blood; also called mono	मोनोन्युक्लियोसिस
mood swing (n)	shift in emotional state, such as happy then sad	मनस्थिति परिवर्तन हुनु
morbidity (n)	1. a diseased condition or state; 2. the incidence of a disease or of all diseases in a population	रोगभार, रोगको प्रकोप
morning sickness (n)	vomiting and nausea that affects some women during the first few weeks of pregnancy, usually occurring in the morning	वाकवाकी
mortuary (n)	a place, esp. a funeral home, where dead bodies are kept prior to burial or cremation	मुर्दाघर
mouth (n)	the body opening through which a human takes in food	मुख
mouthwash (n)	a flavored liquid for cleaning the mouth and making one's breath smell better	माउथवास

English-Nepali Medical Glossary – M

Term	Definition	Nepali
mucous membrane (n)	the moist membrane lining all bodily channels that communicate with the air, such as the respiratory and digestive tracts, the glands of which secrete mucus	श्लेष्म झिल्ली
mucus (n)	the free slime of the mucous membranes, composed of secretion of the glands, along with various inorganic salts	श्लेष्म
multidose (n)	occurring in, or using more than one dose	बहुमात्रा
multiparous (adj)	having had one or more previous successful pregnancies	बहुबेते
multiple sclerosis (n)	a degenerative disease of the central nervous system resulting in weakness and a variety of neurological symptoms	मल्टिपल स्केलेरोसीस
mumps (n)	an acute, inflammatory, contagious disease of the glands that produce saliva	हाँडेरोग
muscle (n)	a tissue in the body comprised of fibers which can tighten and relax to produce movement	मांसपेशी
muscle relaxant (n)	an agent that specifically aids in reducing muscle tension	मांसपेशीलाई आराम दिने
muscular (adj)	of, or pertaining to muscle	मांसपेशीको
muscular system (n)	the organization and action of muscles in the body that control movement, aid digestion, and help blood circulation	मांसपेशी प्रणाली
mute (adj)	unable to speak	मूक
mycosis (n)	any disease caused by a fungus	ढुसीजन्य रोग
myeloma (n)	a tumor composed of cells of the type normally found in the bone marrow	हाडको मासीको क्यान्सार

Term	Definition	Nepali
myocardial infarction (n)	heart attack	मायोकारडीयल इनफार्कसन
myopia (n)	a condition in which the eye does not focus properly on distant objects without the aid of glasses; nearsightedness	निकट दृष्टि

English-Nepali Medical Glossary – N

Term	Definition	Nepali
narcotic (n)	any natural or synthetic drug that has morphine-like actions; a painkiller	मादक
nasal (adj)	of, or pertaining to the nose	नाकको
nasal congestion (n)	a condition where excess mucus in the nose makes breathing difficult	नाक बन्द हुनु
nasal irrigation (n)	a procedure where the nasal canal is cleaned with a liquid to treat disease or an infection	नाकमा तरल पदार्थ हाल्नु
nasal polyp (n)	a growth found in the tissue of the nose	नाकमा मासु पलाउनु
nausea (n)	an unpleasant sensation often including vomiting and upset stomach	वाकवाकी
nauseated (adj)	affected with nausea, the state of having an unpleasant sensation often including vomiting and upset stomach	वाकवाकी लाग्नु
nauseous (adj)	of, or pertaining to the feelings of nausea	वाकवाकी लागेको अवस्था
navel (n)	the mark left on the abdomen where the umbilical cord was attached; belly button	नाभि
nearsighted (adj)	unable to see distant objects clearly	निकट दृष्टि
neck (n)	the part of the body joining the head to the trunk	घाँटी
needle aspiration biopsy (n)	a procedure involving the removal of fluid from any tissue of the body with a needle or aspiration device, used in diagnosis of a disease	निडल एस्पाईरेसन बायोप्सी
needle, syringe (n)	a medical instrument used to inject fluids into the body or draw them from it	सूई, सियो

English-Nepali Medical Glossary – N

Term	Definition	Nepali
negative (adj)	not affirming the presence of the organism or condition in question; lacking the quality of being positive	नकारात्मक
neonatal (adj)	of, or pertaining to the first four weeks after birth	नवजात
neonatologist (n)	a physician who specializes in the care and treatment of infants within the first 28 days of birth	शिशु विशेषज्ञ
neoplasm (n)	an abnormal new growth of tissue; tumor	क्यान्सर
nephritis (n)	inflammation of the kidney	मृगौलाको सुजन
nephrologist (n)	a physician whose specializes in the study of the kidneys	मृगौला विशेषज्ञ
nephrology (n)	the medical study of the structure and function of the kidneys	मृगौलाशास्त्र
nerve (n)	any of the bundles of fibers capable of sending both sensory and motor signals from one part of the body to another; a fiber that enables movement and feeling	स्नायु
nervous (adj)	of, or pertaining to a nerve or the activity of a nerve	स्नायुको
nervous system (n)	the network of nerves, extending throughout the body, that control movement, feeling, etc.	स्नायु प्रणाली
nervousness (n)	excessive excitability and irritability, with mental and physical unrest	आत्तिएको अवस्था
neurologist (n)	a person who studies the medical science of the nervous system and its disorders	स्नायुरोग विशेषज्ञ
neurology (n)	the medical science of the nervous system and its disorders	तंत्रिका विज्ञान
neuropathy (n)	any and all disease or malfunction of the nerves	स्नायुरोग

English-Nepali Medical Glossary – N

Term	Definition	Nepali
neurosis (n)	any of various functional disorders of the mind or emotions without obvious damage or change to the brain	न्युरोसिस
neurosurgery (n)	surgery of any part of the nervous system	न्यूरोसर्जरी
neurotic (adj)	a person with excessive worries	विक्षिप्त
neurotoxic (adj)	poisonous or destructive to nerve tissue	न्युरोटक्सिक
neutral (adj) (m)	1. not allied with, supporting, or favoring either side; indifferent; 2. not acidic or basic	तटस्थ
neutralization (n)	an act or process of neutralizing	निराकरण
next of kin (n)	the person most closely related to a person	नजिकको नातेदार
nicotine patch (n)	a patch worn on the skin that helps reduce the addiction to tobacco	निकोटिन प्याच
nicotine replacement aids (n)	a nicotine-replacement aid placed in a smoker's mouth to help reduce the habit of using tobacco; the nicotine in the gum passes through the mucous membranes of the mouth	निकोटिन रिप्लेसमेन्ट एड्स
night blindness (n)	the inability to see in the dark	रतन्धो
nipple (n)	the small projection near the center of the mammary gland or breast containing outlets of milk ducts	स्तनको मुन्टो
nitroglycerin (n)	medication used to open blood vessels	नाइट्रोग्लिसरीन
nocturnal (adj)	occurring at, or active at night	रात्रिको
nodule (n)	a small node, as of body tissue; a localized swelling	दाना

English-Nepali Medical Glossary – N

Term	Definition	Nepali
non-contagious (adj)	not able to be spread from person to person	नसर्ने
non-medical home equipment (n)	assistive devices, appliances & supplies which are necessary to assure the client's health, safety and independence	गैर-चिकित्सा गृह उपकरण
non-medical transportation (n)	transportation of members by passenger car, taxicabs, or other forms of public or private conveyances	गैर-चिकित्सा परिवहन
Non-Physician Medical Practitioners (Mid-Level Practitioner) (n)	a nurse practitioner, nurse midwife, or physician assistant allowed to provide primary care under physician supervision	नन-फिजिसियन मेडिकल प्राक्टिसनर (मिड-लेभल प्राक्टिसनर)
nonspecific (adj)	not due to any single known cause	गैर-विशिष्ठ
non-stress test (n)	a test to evaluate fetal well-being by evaluating fetal heart rate response to fetal movement	गैर-तनाव परीक्षण
normal (adj)	usual, standard, or typical	सामान्य
nose (n)	the structure of the face or forward part of the head that contains the organs of smell and forms the beginning of the respiratory tract	नाक
nose drops (n)	a medication administered in drops into the nose	नाकको झोल औषधि
nose spray (n)	a medication administered as a mist into the nose	नाकको स्प्रे
nosebleed (n)	bleeding from the nose	नाथ्री फुट्नु
nostril (n)	either of the external openings of the nose	नाकको प्वाल
nothing by mouth (n)	an instruction by a physician to not eat or drink, usually for a number of hours prior to surgery, or in preparation for a diagnostic test	मुखबाट केहि पनि नलिने

Term	Definition	Nepali
numb (adj)	lacking the power to feel pain or touch	निदाएको, अचेतन
nurse (v)	to feed with milk from the breast; to suckle	स्याहारसुसार गर्नु
nurse practitioner (n)	a registered nurse who can work independently of a physician and provide all levels of care to patients, including treatments and prescriptions	परिचारिका
nursing home (n)	a private hospital for the care of the aged or chronically ill	नर्सिङ होम
nutrient (n)	an important substance for function of the body; food, or a component of food	पोषक तत्व
nutrition (n)	the process of nourishing or being nourished, esp. the process by which humans digest food and use it for growth and for replacement of tissue	पोषण
nutritional supplement (n)	a product intended for ingestion to add to or to complete a diet and that contains one or more of the following dietary ingredients: a vitamin, mineral, amino acid, herb or other botanical	पोषणयुक्त खुराक
nutritionist (n)	a person who specializes in the study of nutrition	पोषणविद्

English-Nepali Medical Glossary – O

Term	Definition	Nepali
obese (adj)	extremely fat; overweight	मोटे, भुंडे
obesity (n)	an increase in body weight; an excessive accumulation of fat in the body	मोटोपना
observation (n)	the act of watching attentively	अवलोकन
obstetric nurse (n)	a nurse specialized in caring for pregnant women	प्रसूति नर्स
obstetrician (n)	a physician specializing in obstetrics	प्रसूति विज्ञ
obstetrics (n)	branch of medicine that deals with pregnancy, childbirth, and the post-partum period	प्रसूति
obstruction (n)	act of blocking or clogging	बाधा
occipital (adj)	of, or pertaining to the back of the head, esp. the posterior part of the skull	पश्चकपाल
occult (adj)	hidden from view; concealed from observation; difficult to understand	लुकेको, छोपिएको
occult blood (n)	blood that cannot be seen, but is identified by using special techniques, usually referring to blood in the stool	नदेखिएको रगत
occupational disease (n)	a disease caused by work-related activities	पेशागत रोग
ocular (adj)	of, or pertaining to the eye; seen by the eye	आँखाको
oculist (n)	a physician who treats disease of the eyes; ophthalmologist	नेत्र विशेषज्ञ
oil (n)	any of numerous mineral, vegetable, and man-made substances and animal and vegetable fats that are generally slippery, inflammable, and liquid at room temperatures	तेल

Term	Definition	Nepali
ointment (n)	a medication applied to the skin	मलम
on an empty stomach (prep)	describing a physical state of not having eaten for an extended period, thereby having digested all the food in the stomach	खालि पेटमा
oncologist (n)	a physician who specializes in the study of cancer	क्यान्सर विशेषज्ञ
onset (n)	the beginning, esp. of an illness	सुरु
ooze (v)	to flow or leak out slowly, as through small openings	चुहिनु, रसाउनु
operate (v) (m)	to perform surgery	शल्यक्रिया गर्नु
operating room (n)	a section of a hospital where surgical procedures are performed	शल्यक्रिया कक्ष
operation (n) (m)	a procedure for repairing or relieving an injury, ailment, or dysfunction in a living body, esp. performed with instruments; surgery	शल्यक्रिया
ophthalmic (adj)	pertaining to the eye	आँखाको
ophthalmologic (adj)	of, or pertaining to the branch of medicine dealing with the eye	नेत्र विज्ञानको
ophthalmologist (n)	a physician who specializes in the anatomy, functions, pathology, and treatment of the eye	नेत्र विशेषज्ञ
ophthalmology (n)	the branch of medicine dealing with the eye	नेत्र विज्ञान
opiate (n)	a remedy containing or derived from opium; also any drug that induces sleep or relieves pain	अफिमयुक्त
optic (adj)	of, or pertaining to the eye	आँखाको
optic nerve (n)	the nerve that delivers signals from the eye to the brain	आँखाको स्नायु
optimal (adj)	the best; the most favorable	ठिक मात्रामा

Term	Definition	Nepali
optometrist (n)	a person whose profession is examining, measuring, and treating certain visual defects by means of corrective lenses or other methods that do not require a physician's license	ओप्टोमेट्रीस्ट
optometry (n)	the profession of examining, measuring, and treating certain visual defects by means of corrective lenses or other methods that do not require license as a physician	ओप्टोमेट्री
oral (adj)	1. pertaining to the mouth (adj); 2. taken through or applied in the mouth (adv)	मुखको
oral cavity (n)	the mouth	मुख
oral surgery (n)	surgery specific to the mouth	मुखको शल्यक्रिया
organ (n)	a differentiated part of the human, adapted for a specific function, such as the heart or lungs	अंग
organ donor (n)	a person who gives an organ to another patient	अंग दाता
orthodontist (n)	a dentist who specializes in the practice of correcting abnormally aligned or positioned teeth	दन्त विशेषज्ञ
orthopedics (n)	the study of the musculoskeletal system	हाडजोर्नीको अध्ययन
orthopedist (n)	a physician who specializes in the surgical or manipulative treatment of disorders of the skeletal system and associated motor organs	हाडजोर्नी विशेषज्ञ
ossicle (n)	a small ear bone	सानो हड्डी
osteoarthritis (n)	degenerative joint disease	ऑस्टियोआर्थराइटिस

English-Nepali Medical Glossary – O

Term	Definition	Nepali
osteoporosis (n)	reduction in the amount of bone mass, leading to fractures after minimal trauma	ऑस्टियोपोरोसिस
osteotomy (n)	the surgical cutting of a bone	हड्डी काटेर हटाउने
otitis (n)	inflammation of the ear, which may be marked by pain, fever, abnormalities of hearing, etc.	कानको सुजन
otoscope (n)	a device used to examine the ear	ओटोस्कोप
outer ear (n)	the portion of the ear that consists of the auricle and ear canal	बाहिरि कान
outpatient (n)	a patient who receives treatment at a hospital or clinic without being hospitalized	बहिरंग बिरामी
ovarian (adj)	pertaining to an ovary or ovaries	डिम्बासयको
ovarian cyst (n)	a cyst that has grown on or originated from an ovary	डिम्बासयको फुकुन्डो
ovary (n)	one of a pair of female reproductive glands located on both sides of the uterus	डिम्बासय
over the counter (drugs) (prep/n)	medication that can be purchased without a prescription	पुर्जा बिनानै किन्न सकिने (औषधि)
overactive thyroid (n)	hyperthyroidism; excessive production of thyroid hormone	अति सक्रिय थाईरोइड
overdosage (n)	administration of an excessive dose; condition resulting from an excessive dose	मात्र भन्दा बढी दिइनु
overdose (n)	an excessive dose	मात्रा भन्दा बढी
ovulation (n)	the period during a woman's monthly cycle where a mature egg is released, making her very susceptible to pregnancy	डिम्बोत्सर्जन
oxygen (n)	a colorless, odorless, tasteless gaseous element essential for respiration and essential for human life	अक्सिजन

Term	Definition	Nepali
oxygenation (n)	process of supplying, treating, or mixing with oxygen	अक्सिजनयुक्त बनाउने काम

English-Nepali Medical Glossary – P

Term	Definition	Nepali
pacemaker (n)	a device which influences the rate of the heart	पेसमेकर
pain (n)	an unpleasant sensation, occurring in varying degrees of severity as a consequence of injury, disease, or emotional disorder	पिडा
pain, constant (n)	pain that continues without subsiding	लगातारको पिडा
pain, dull (n)	pain that is not intensely or keenly felt	हल्का पिडा
pain killer (n)	something, such as a drug, that relieves pain	पिडा निवारक
pain, on and off (n)	pain that is felt and then is not felt	यदाकदा हुने पिडा
pain, radiating (n)	discomfort that originates from a central location and spreads outward, esp. down the arm and shoulder	फैलेको पिडा
pain, sharp (n)	pain that is harsh or biting	कडा पिडा
pain, shooting (n)	a sudden intense feeling of pain or discomfort	एक्कासी भएको पिडा
pain, throbbing (n)	pain that vibrates, pulsates, or has a rhythm	बल्किएको पिडा
painful (adj)	causing pain; hurtful	पीडायुक्त
palate (n)	the roof of the mouth consisting of a bony front, the hard palate, backed by the fleshy soft palate	तालू
pale (adj)	whitish, referring to skin color	रक्तबिहिन, फुङ्ग
palliative (adj)	of, or pertaining to medical treatment affording relief, but no cure	पिडा कम गर्ने
pallor (n)	extreme or unnatural paleness	एकदमै फुङ्ग हुनु
palm (n)	the inner surface of the hand, extending from the wrist to the base of the fingers	हत्केला

English-Nepali Medical Glossary – P

Term	Definition	Nepali
palpitation (n)	a rapid or irregular heart beat; the act of shaking, quivering, or fluttering	मुटु काम्नु, आत्तिनु
pamphlet (n)	a piece of folded paper printed with information about a procedure, program, disease, or health issue	पम्पेल्ट, पुस्तिका
pancreas (n)	a long, soft, irregularly shaped gland lying behind the stomach that helps with digestion and metabolism	पेंक्रियाज
pancreatitis (n)	acute or chronic inflammation of the pancreas	पेंक्रियाजको सुजन
pap smear, pap test (n)	a procedure in which cells are collected from the cervix and examined for cancer	प्याप स्मियर, प्याप परीक्षण
paralysis (n)	loss or impairment of motor function	पक्षघात
paramedic (n)	a person who is trained to supply emergency medical treatment or to assist medical professionals	चिकित्सकको सहायक
paranoia (n)	a very unstable mental condition in which the person has a feeling of being in danger, chased, or threatened	विक्षिप्त
paraplegia (n)	paralysis of the legs and lower part of the body	तल्लो भागको पक्षघात
parasite (n)	an organism that grows, feeds, and lives on or in another organism, usually causing harm to the other organism	परजीवी
parasitic (adj)	of, or pertaining to, or caused by a parasite	परजीवी जन्य
parathyroid (n)	one of four glands situated beside the thyroid gland that are involved in hormone secretion	पाराथाईरोइड

English-Nepali Medical Glossary – P

Term	Definition	Nepali
paresthesia (n)	abnormal or impaired skin sensation, such as burning, prickling, itching, or tingling	झमझमाउने
parietal (adj)	1. of, or pertaining to the walls of a cavity; 2. of, or pertaining to a specific portion of the skull	पार्श्वीय
Parkinson's Disease (n)	a progressive nervous disease of older people, characterized by involuntary movements, partial facial paralysis, difficulty walking, and general weakness	पार्किन्सन डिजिज
partner (n)	one associated with another, especially in an action	साथी
pass out (v)	to become unconscious, without awareness, and not capable of voluntary movement	बेहोस हुनु
pasta (n)	a food, such as spaghetti, made from water and flour and formed into different shapes then cooked in boiling water; it is high in carbohydrates	पास्ता
patella (n)	kneecap; a flat, triangular bone located at the front of the knee joint	घुँडाको पाँग्रा
pathogen (n)	any disease-producing microorganism	रोगाणु
pathogenic (adj)	capable of causing a disease	रोगजनक
pathologic (adj)	pathological; of, or pertaining to pathology; pertaining to or caused by disease	रोगाणु सम्बन्धित
pathologist (n)	a person who specializes in the study of pathology	रोगविज्ञ
pathology (n)	the scientific study of the nature of disease, its causes, processes, development, and consequences	रोग विज्ञान
patient (n)	person receiving medical treatment	बिरामी

English-Nepali Medical Glossary – P

Term	Definition	Nepali
patient advocate (n)	a person who argues for a patient, who supports a patient in gaining equal access to health care (this is different than an interpreter taking on the advocate role, which is an action an interpreter takes on behalf of the patient outside the bounds of an interpreted interview)	बिरामीको अधिवक्ता
peak-flow meter (n)	a hand-held device that measures air flow (how fast air is blown out of the lungs); patients can use peak-flow meters to measure their own air flow regularly	पीक फ्लो मीटर
pediatric nurse practitioner (n)	a registered nurse with advanced training who provides primary health care to children	बाल चिकित्सा नर्स
pediatrician (n)	a physician who specializes in the care and medical treatment of children	बाल चिकित्सक
pediatrics (n)	care and medical treatment of children	बाल रोग
pelvic (adj)	of, or pertaining to the pelvis	नितम्बको
pelvic inflammatory disease (n)	infection of the uterus and adjacent pelvic structures	नितम्बको सुजनहुने रोग
pelvis (n)	a basin-shaped skeletal structure that rests on the bones of the lower limbs and supports the spinal column	नितम्ब
penetration (n)	act of piercing or entering deeply	प्रवेश
penis (n)	male organ of sexual intercourse and of urinary excretion	लिङ्ग
peptic (adj)	of, or pertaining to, or assisting digestion	पाचन सम्बन्धि

English-Nepali Medical Glossary – P

Term	Definition	Nepali
peptic ulcer disease (n)	a hole in the lining of the stomach, duodenum, or esophagus; a peptic ulcer occurs when the lining of these organs is corroded by the acidic digestive juices that are secreted by the stomach cells	पेप्टिक अल्सर रोग
percutaneous (adj)	performed through the skin, as injection	छाला मार्फत
perforation (n)	act of boring or piercing through a part	प्वाल, छिद्र
perinatal (adj)	pertaining to or occurring in the period shortly before and after birth	प्रसवकालीन
perineum (n)	the portion of the body in the pelvis occupied by the bladder, uterus, ovaries, rectum, etc., bounded in front by the pubic arch, in back by the tailbone, and to the sides by the hipbone	मलद्वार र मुत्रद्वारको बिचको भाग
period (menstrual) (n) (m)	an instance or occurrence of menstruation	महिनावारि
period (related to time) (n) (m)	an interval of time characterized by the occurrence of certain conditions or events	अवधी
periodontal disease (n)	a disease of the tissue and structures surrounding and supporting the teeth	दाँत वरिपरिको तन्तुको रोग
periosteum (n)	the fibrous membrane covering bone that supports blood vessels and the attachment of ligaments, tendons, and muscles	हड्डीको झिल्ली
persistent (adj)	continuing to exist in spite of interference or treatment; tending to recur	लगातार
personal care (adj)	provides assistance to maintain bodily hygiene, personal safety, and activities of daily living	व्यक्तिगत रेखदेख

English-Nepali Medical Glossary – P

Term	Definition	Nepali
perspiration (n)	sweating; the functional secretion of sweat	पसीना
perspire (v)	to excrete sweat or perspiration through the pores of the skin	पसीना निकाल्नु
pertussis (n)	an acute, highly contagious infection of the respiratory tract, causing a harsh cough; most frequently affecting young children	लहरेखोकी
pessary (n)	instrument placed in the vagina to support the uterus or rectum or as a device to prevent pregnancy	पेसरी
phallic (adj)	pertaining to the penis	लैङ्गिक
pharmacist (n)	a person trained in pharmacy; druggist	औषधि विक्रेता
pharmacy (n)	a place where medicines are prepared and sold	औषधालय
pharynx (n)	the section of throat that allows for the passage of air and the passage of food	कण्ठ
phlebitis (n)	inflammation of a vein	शिराको सुजन
phlegm (n)	stringy, thick mucus	कफ
phobia (n)	persistent, irrational, intense fear of a specific object, activity, or situation	भय
photophobia (n)	abnormal visual intolerance of light	प्रकाश असहनसिलता
physical (adj)	pertaining to the body, to material things, or to physics	शारीरिक
physical exam (n)	a general examination of the body for any diseases, disorders, or pathogenic conditions	शारीरिक परीक्षा
physical therapist (n)	a person trained to treat disease and injury by mechanical means, such as exercise, heat, light, and massage	शारीरिक चिकित्सक

English-Nepali Medical Glossary – P

Term	Definition	Nepali
physical therapy (n)	the treatment of disease and injury by mechanical means, such as exercise, heat, light, and massage	शारीरिक चिकित्सा
physician (n)	doctor; a person trained in the healing arts and licensed to practice	चिकित्सक
physician's assistant (n)	a person trained to assist a physician in procedures and examination of patients	चिकित्सकको सहायक
pigment (n)	a substance used as coloring	रंग
pigmentation (n)	coloration of tissues by pigment	रंग चड्नु
piles (n)	hemorrhoids	रगतयुक्त दिसा
pill (n)	a small pellet or tablet of medicine, often coated, taken by swallowing whole or chewing	चक्की, गोलि
pillow (n)	a soft stuffed cloth cushion used to rest the head, esp. during sleep	सिरानी
pimple (n)	a small swelling of the skin, sometimes containing pus	डण्डीफोर
pituitary gland (n)	a small, oval endocrine gland attached to the base of the brain that controls growth, maturation, and metabolism	पिट्यूटरी ग्रंथि
placebo (n)	a medication or treatment known to have no effect, often used for comparison in an experiment	प्लासिबो
placenta (n)	an organ located in the uterus that joins a mother to her unborn baby and through which it receives nourishment	सालनाल
plague (n)	a highly infectious, usually fatal, epidemic disease	प्लेग, महामारी
plasma (n)	the liquid part of blood	प्लाज्मा

English-Nepali Medical Glossary – P

Term	Definition	Nepali
plastic surgery (n)	surgery to remodel, repair, or restore injured or defective body parts, esp. by transfer of tissue	प्लास्टिक सर्जरी
platelets (n)	a disk, smaller than a red blood cell, found in the blood, which helps prevent bleeding	प्लेटलेट्स
pleura (n)	either of two sacs, each of which lines one side of the chest cavity and holds the lungs	फोक्सोको खोल, प्लुरा
pleural cavity (n)	the space within the pleura where the lungs are located	प्लुराले बनाएको खाली ठाउँ
pleural effusion (n)	the escape of fluid from the blood vessels in the pleural cavity	प्लुराको चुहावट
pleural rub (n)	friction of one surface moving over another causing inflammation of the pleural cavity	प्लुराको घर्षण
pleurisy (n)	inflammation of the pleural cavity	प्लुराको सुजन
plugged ear (n)	a condition in which there is a clot, usually of ear wax, in the ear canal, causing difficulties in hearing	कान टालीनु
pneumococcal pneumonia (n)	lung infection caused by Streptococcus pneumoniae	न्यूमोकोकल निमोनिया
pneumonia (n)	inflammation of the lungs caused by virus, bacteria, and physical and chemical agents	निमोनिया
pneumothorax (n)	accumulation of air or gas in the pleural cavity, occurring as a result of disease or injury	वातवक्ष
podiatrist (n)	a person whose profession is the study and treatment of foot problems	खुट्टा विशेषज्ञ
poison (n)	a substance that causes injury, illness, or death, esp. by chemical means	बिष

English-Nepali Medical Glossary – P

Term	Definition	Nepali
policy (n)	a plan or course of action; guiding principle or procedure considered to be expedient, prudent, or advantageous	नीति
polio (n)	poliomyelitis; an acute viral disease, occurring sporadically and in epidemics, which causes paralysis	पोलियो
pollen (n)	small, light, dry protein particles from trees, grasses, flowers, and weeds that may be spread by the wind; pollen is a potent stimulator of allergic responses	पराग
pollutant (n)	something that pollutes, esp. a waste material that contaminates air, soil, or water	प्रदूषक
pollute (v)	to make unfit for or harmful to humans, animals and plants, esp. by the addition of waste matter or harmful chemicals	प्रदुषित पार्नु
pollution (n)	the act or process of polluting or the state of being polluted; the contamination of the body by the exposure to harmful substances	प्रदूषण
polyp (n)	a growth protruding from the mucous lining of an organ such as the nose	मासु पलाउनु
pores (n)	very small openings	छिद्र
positive (adj)	indicating a presence of a particular disease, condition, or organism	सकारात्मक
post nasal drip (n)	the chronic secretion of mucus from the posterior nasal cavities, resulting in soreness and congestion of the throat	गलामा सिंगान झर्नु

English-Nepali Medical Glossary – P

Term	Definition	Nepali
posterior (adj)	situated in back of, or in the back part of, or affecting the back or dorsal surface of the body	पछाडिको
postmenopausal (adj)	occurring after menopause	रजनोवृत्ति पछिको
postnatal (adj)	occurring after birth, with reference to the newborn	सुत्केरी भएपछिको
postoperative (adj)	occurring after a surgical operation	शल्यक्रिया पछिको
post-partum (adj)	of, or occurring in the period shortly after childbirth	प्रसव पछिको
post-traumatic (adj)	occurring as a result of or after injury	चोट पश्चात
posture (n)	a position or attitude of the body or of bodily parts	मुद्रा
pound (n)	a unit of weight equal to 16 ounces	पाउण्ड (तौल)
power of attorney (n)	a legal instrument authorizing one to act as another's attorney or agent	वकिलको शक्ति
preclinical (adj)	before a disease becomes recognizable to a doctor	लक्षण देखिनु पूर्वको
preeclampsia (n)	development of high blood pressure due to pregnancy or the influence of a recent pregnancy	प्रीएक्लाम्पसिया
pregnancy (n)	the condition of being pregnant	गर्भावस्था
pregnancy test (n)	a procedure used to determine if someone is pregnant	गर्भावस्था परीक्षण
pregnant (adj)	carrying a developing baby within the uterus	गर्भवती
preload (n)	the load of blood waiting to get into the heart	पूर्वभार, प्रिलोड
premature (adj)	occurring before the proper time, esp. a premature infant	अपरिपक्व
pre-menstrual (adj)	occurring before menstruation	महिनावारी पूर्व
prenatal (adj)	existing or occurring before birth, with reference to the baby	जन्म पूर्व

English-Nepali Medical Glossary – P

Term	Definition	Nepali
prenatal care (n)	medical care given to the mother prior to birth	प्रसव पूर्व रेखदेख
pre-operative (adj)	preceding an operation	शल्यक्रिया पूर्वको
presbyopia (n)	the inability of the eye to focus sharply on nearby objects, usually occurring with advancing age	दीर्घचक्षु
prescribe (v)	to order or recommend the use of a drug or treatment	औषधि दिनु
prescription (n)	a written direction for the preparation and administration of a remedy	औषधि पुर्जा
pressure (n)	the act of applying a continuous force on something	चाप, थिचाई
pressure sore (n)	bed sore	थिचाईले बनाउने घाउ
preteen (n)	child of age group 10 to 12 years old	१०-१२ बर्षको
prevent (v)	to keep from happening	रोक्नु
preventative (adj)	designed or used to prevent or hinder; thwarting or warding off illness or disease	निवारक
preventive care services (n)	services provided to prevent illness; there are three (3) levels of preventive care: primary, such as immunizations, aimed at preventing disease; secondary, such as disease screening programs, aimed at early detection of disease; and tertiary, such as physical therapy, aimed at restoring function after the disease has occurred	निवारक रेखदेख सेवा
prick (v)	to puncture or poke lightly	घोचाइ

Term	Definition	Nepali
primary care physician (PCP) (n)	a physician who focuses his/her practice of medicine on general practice or who is a board certified or board eligible internist, pediatrician, obstetrician/gynecologist, or family practitioner; this physician is responsible for supervising, coordinating, and providing initial and primary care	प्राथमिक उपचार चिकित्सक
primary care provider (n)	a person or other health care provider responsible for supervising, coordinating, and providing initial and primary care to patients; this provider is responsible for initiating referrals and maintaining the continuity of patient care	प्राथमिक उपचार प्रदायक
primary care services (n)	a physician or other health care provider who does not specialize in a particular area but treats a variety of medical problems, usually serving a family	प्राथमिक उपचार सेवाहरु
primary vaccination (n)	first or principal vaccination	प्राथमिक खोपकार्य
prior authorization review (n)	the process of obtaining prior approval from one's health insurance provider as to the appropriateness of a service or medication; prior authorization does not guarantee insurance coverage	पूर्व प्राधिकरणको समीक्षा
procreation (n)	entire process of bringing a new individual into the world	जन्माउनु

English-Nepali Medical Glossary – P

Term	Definition	Nepali
prognosis (n)	a forecast as to the probable outcome of an illness or injury; the prospect as to recovery from a disease as indicated by the nature and symptons of the case	पूर्वानुमान
program (n)	a plan or system under which action may be taken toward a goal	योजना
progressive (adj)	advancing; going forward; increasing in scope or severity	प्रगतिशील
prolapse (n)	the falling down, or sinking of an organ or part, such as a prolapse of the uterus	खस्नु
proliferation (n)	reproduction or multiplication of similar forms	प्रसार
prophylaxis (n)	prevention of disease; preventive treatment	रोकथाम
prostate gland (n)	a gland in males composed of muscular and glandular tissue that surrounds the urethra at the bladder	प्रोस्टेट ग्रंथि
prosthesis (n)	an artificial replacement of a missing part of the body, esp. an arm or leg	कृत्रिम अंग
protective supervision (n)	insures provision of 24 hour supervision to persons in their homes who are very frail or otherwise may suffer a medical emergency, to prevent immediate placement in an acute care hospital, skilled nursing facility, or other 24–hour care facility	सुरक्षात्मक पर्यवेक्षण
protein (n) (m)	an essential nutrient for growth and survival of the human body	प्रोटीन

English-Nepali Medical Glossary – P

Term	Definition	Nepali
provider (of health care) (n)	a physician, nurse, technician, teacher, hospital, insurance company, health maintenance organization, voluntary agency, or other person or institution engaged in furnishing some type of care to individuals	प्रदायक (स्वास्थ्यसेवा)
pruritus (n)	severe itching, usually of undamaged skin	अत्याधिक चिलाउनु
psoriasis (n)	a chronic, non-contagious skin disease characterized by inflammation and white, scaly patches	पाप्रा हुने
psychiatrist (n)	a physician who specializes in the study, diagnosis, treatment, and prevention of mental illness	मनोचिकित्सक
psychologist (n)	a non-physician who specializes in the study of mental processes and behavior	मनोवैज्ञानिक
psychology (n)	the science of mental processes and behavior	मनोविज्ञान
puberty (n)	the stage of life when an individual becomes capable of sexual reproduction	यौवन
pubic bone (n)	a bone found in the pelvis below the abdomen	जाँघको हड्डी
pubic hair (n)	the hair growing around the external genitals	जाँघको रौँ
pubis (n)	the area over the pubic bone, below the abdomen	जाँघ
pulmonary abscess (n)	a pus-containing infection in the lung	फोक्सोमा पिप जम्ने
pulmonary angiography (n)	a procedure that examines the blood vessels in the lungs by injecting a substance into the blood vessel and taking an x-ray image	पल्मोनरी एन्जिओग्राफि

English-Nepali Medical Glossary – P

Term	Definition	Nepali
pulmonary artery (n)	an artery that supplies blood to the lungs	फोक्सोको धमनी
pulmonary edema (n)	the presence of excess fluid in the lungs	फोक्सोमा पानी भरिने
pulmonary embolism (n)	the obstruction of a blood vessel in a lung	फोक्सोको नसाहरुको रोकावट
pulmonary function tests (n)	one of a number of tests used to determine the ability of the lungs to exchange oxygen and carbon dioxide	फोक्सोको कार्य परिक्षण
pulmonary infarction (n)	a condition where blood cannot be delivered to the lungs; it is usually caused by a blood clot	फोक्सोको रोधगलन
pulmonologist (n)	a physician who specializes in the treatment and study of lung diseases	फोक्सोको विशेषज्ञ
pulse (n)	the throbbing of arteries produced by the regular contractions of the heart	नाडी
pump the stomach (v)	a medical procedure used to remove all contents of the stomach in an effort to remove toxic substances	पेट खाली गर्नु
pupil (of eye) (n) (m)	the apparently black circular area in the center of the eye	नानी (आँखाको)
purified protein derivative (n)	a test administered by injection to determine if a patient has tuberculosis	प्युरीफाइड प्रोटिन डेरीभेटिभ
purulent (adj)	containing or secreting pus	पीपयुक्त
pus (n)	a yellowish-white fluid, consisting mainly of white blood cells and cellular debris, that forms in infected tissue	पीप

Term	Definition	Nepali
push (v)	to exert force against an object to move it away; to move an object by exerting force against it; to thrust; to shove; to bear hard upon; to press	धकाल्नु
pustule (n)	a slight, inflamed, pus-filled elevation of the skin	पीपयुक्त पिड्का

English-Nepali Medical Glossary – Q

Term	Definition	Nepali
quadriceps (n)	a large four-part muscle on the front of the leg between the knee and hip	चारकुने मांसपेशी
Qualified Medicare Beneficiary (QMB) (n)	a person whose income falls below 100% of federal poverty guidelines, for whom the state must pay the Medicare Part B premiums, deductibles, and co-payments	क्वालिफाइड मेडीकेयर बेनिफिसीयरी (क्यु.एम.बि.)
quality of care (n)	the degree or grade of excellence with respect to medical services received by enrollees, administered by providers or programs, in terms of technical competence, needs appropriateness, acceptability, humanity, structure, etc	रेखदेखको गुणस्तर
quarantine (n)	a period of time during which a vehicle, a person, or material suspected of carrying a contagious disease is detained; enforced isolation or restriction of free movement imposed to prevent a contagious disease from spreading	निषेधावधी
queasy (adj)	1. uneasy; 2. having an upset stomach; nauseated; sickening	पेट बिगार्ने
quiescent (adj)	marked by a state of inactivity or repose	मौन

English-Nepali Medical Glossary – R

Term	Definition	Nepali
rabies (n)	an acute, infectious, often fatal viral disease of most warm-blooded animals, esp. wolves, cats, and dogs, that attacks the central nervous system and is transmitted by the bite of the infected animal	रेबीज
radiation (n)	beams of energy used to make x-rays, or to kill cancer cells	विकिरण
radioactive (adj)	being capable of releasing radiation	रेडियोधर्मी
radioactive iodine (n)	iodine that emits radiation and is used in medical procedures to generate images of the internal structures of the body, usually the thyroid gland	रेडियोधर्मी आयोडिन
radiologist (n)	a physician who specializes in the use of ionizing radiation for medical diagnosis, esp. the use of x-rays in medical imaging	रेडियोलोजीस्ट
radiology technician (n)	a person trained to maintain and operate x-ray or radiography equipment	रेडियोलोजी प्राविधिक
radius (n)	the outer, shorter bone of the forearm	अर्धव्यास
rales, crackles (n)	abnormal sounds during breathing	घुराइ
range of motion exercises (n)	a measure of one's flexibility and capabilities in movement, usually examined after an injury	गति व्यायामहरु
rape (v)	the crime of forcing another person to submit to sexual intercourse	बलात्कार
rash (n) (m)	a skin eruption	बिबिरा
razor (n)	a sharp-edged cutting instrument	छुरा

English-Nepali Medical Glossary – R

Term	Definition	Nepali
reactive (n)	tending to be responsive or to react to a stimulus	प्रतिक्रियाशील
reading glasses (n)	glasses worn to assist in focusing while reading	पढ्ने चश्मा
reagent (n)	substance used to detect other substances, used in laboratory testing	रिएजेन्ट
receptionist (n)	an office worker employed chiefly to receive visitors and answer the telephone	रिसेप्शनिस्ट
recipient (n)	a person who has been designated by a Medicaid agency as eligible to receive Medicaid benefits (sometimes referred to as beneficiary)	प्राप्तकर्ता
recommended (v)	endorsed as fit, worthy, or competent	सिफारिश गर्नु
reconstitution (n)	the return to an original state of a substance, or combination of parts to make a whole	पुनर्गठन
reconstructive surgery (n)	a surgical procedure that attempts to restore damaged tissue or organs to their original state	पुननिर्माण शल्यक्रिया
records (n) (m)	medical records; an organized database or file that contains the medical history of one or more patients	अभिलेख
recovery room (n)	a hospital room equipped for the care and observation of patients immediately following surgery	स्वास्थ्यलाभ कक्ष
rectal (adj)	pertaining to the rectum	मलाशयको
rectum (n)	the distal or end portion of the large intestine, where stool (feces) is stored prior to defecation	मलाशय

English-Nepali Medical Glossary – R

Term	Definition	Nepali
recuperation (n)	the recovery of health and strength	स्वास्थ्यलाभ
recurrent (adj)	occurring or appearing again or repeatedly	पुनरावर्ती
red blood cell (n)	a red-colored cell capable of transporting oxygen throughout the body	रक्त कोशिका
reduction (n) (m)	the correction of a fracture, dislocation, or hernia, moving it back to its normal location	ठिक पार्ने काम
reflex (n)	an involuntary action or movement	रिफ्लैक्स
reflux (n)	a backward or return flow	पछाडीतिर बग्नु
refractory (adj)	not responsive to treatment	प्रतिरोधी
regeneration (n)	the natural renewal of a structure, as of lost tissue or a part	पुनर्जीवित हुनु
registered nurse (n)	a graduate trained nurse who has passed a state registration examination	पंजीकृत नर्स
registration (n)	the act of officially recording items, names, or actions, or the place where such recording is performed	पंजीकरण
regression (n)	a return to a former or earlier state	प्रतिगमन
regurgitation (n)	a backward flowing, as the casting up of undigested food, or the backward flowing of blood into the heart, or between the chambers of the heart when a valve is not working properly	उकेल्ने कार्य
rehabilitation (n)	the process of restoring a patient, such as a handicapped person, to optimal life through education and therapy	पुनर्वास
rehydration (n)	restoration of water or fluid content to a body	पुनर्जलीकरण

English-Nepali Medical Glossary – R

Term	Definition	Nepali
reinfection (n)	a second infection by the same organism or virus	पुनसंक्रमण
relapse (n)	falling back or reversion to a former state; regression after partial recovery from illness	पुनरावर्तन
relative (n)	a person who is related by marriage, ancestry, or family	नातेदार
relax (v)	to calm, rest, or reduce mobility; to make loose	आराम गर्नु
relaxant (n)	something, such as a drug or therapeutic treatment, that relaxes or relieves muscular or nervous tension	आराम दिने औषधि
relieve (v)	to alleviate or lessen pain or discomfort	राहत दिनु
remedy (n)	something, such as medicine or therapy, that relieves pain, cures disease, or corrects a disorder	उपचार
remission (n)	the condition or period when the symptoms of a disease are not visible	रोगको लक्षण नदेखिएको
remove (v)	to take away; to do away with	हटाउनु
renal (adj)	pertaining to the kidney	मिर्गौलाको
replicate (v)	to duplicate, copy, or repeat	नक्कल गर्नु
reproductive system (n)	the system of organs, glands, tissues, and hormones involved in reproduction	प्रजनन प्रणाली
research (v)	to search or investigate by collecting information	अनुसंधान
resection (n)	the removal of a portion or all of an organ or other structure	शल्यक्रियाद्वारा हटाउने
resident (n) (m)	a physician serving a period of residency, the period during which a physician receives specialized clinical training	निवासी
respiration (n)	the act or process of inhaling and exhaling; breathing	श्वासप्रश्वास

English-Nepali Medical Glossary – R

Term	Definition	Nepali
respiratory system (n)	the integrated system of organs involved in the intake and exchange of oxygen and carbon dioxide between a human and the atmosphere	श्वासप्रश्वास प्रणाली
respite care service (n)	service that provides relief for a patient's caretaker	राहत रेखदेख सेवा
restraints (n)	straps used to restrict movement	अंकुश
resuscitation (n)	the restoration to life or consciousness of one apparently dead	पुनर्जीवन
retardation (n)	delay, slowness in development or progress	मन्दता
retina (n)	the inner layer of the eyeball that responds to light and enables sight by sending signals to the brain	रेटिना
retinal detachment (n)	a condition where the retina cannot send signals to the brain thereby causing blindness	रेटिनल डीट्याचमेन्ट
retinal disease (n)	a disease of the retina of the eye; the retina is weakened by tiny blood vessels of the eye either from small tears or holes, or lack of blood going to these blood vessels, which results in loss of vision	रेटिनाको रोग
retinopathy (n)	a disease or disorder of the retina	रेटिनाको रोग
retraction (n)	1. act of drawing back; 2. reduction of tissue volume	संकुचन
rheumatic fever (n)	a severe infectious disease occurring chiefly in children, characterized by fever and painful inflammation of the joints, and frequently resulting in permanent damage to the valves of the heart	बातज्वरो

English-Nepali Medical Glossary – R

Term	Definition	Nepali
rheumatic heart disease (n)	heart disease caused by rheumatic fever	बात र मुटुरोग
rheumatism (n)	any of several pathological conditions of the muscles, tendons, joints, bones, or nerves, characterized by fever and painful inflammation of the joints	बात
rheumatoid arthritis (n)	a chronic disease marked by stiffness and inflammation of the joints, weakness, loss of mobility, and deformity	बात
rheumatoid factor test (n)	a test that determines whether a rheumatoid factor is present in the blood; the presence of this factor may indicate rheumatoid arthritis	रयुमेटोईड फ्याक्टर टेस्ट
rheumatologist (n)	a physician who studies any of several pathological conditions of the muscles, tendons, joints, bones, or nerves	बात विशेषज्ञ
rhinitis (n)	inflammation of the mucous membrane of the nose	रुघा
rhinoscope (n)	an instrument used to examine the nasal passages	राइनोस्कोप
rhonchus (n)	a snoring sound; a rattling in the throat	घुरेको आवाज
rib (n)	one of a series of long, curved bones, occurring in 12 pairs in human beings and extending from the spine to or toward the sternum or breast plate	करङ
rice (n)	a type of grain (white to brown in color) common in many foods and high in carbohydrates	चामल
rickets (n)	disease marked by bending and distortion of the bones; caused by vitamin D deficiency	बालवक्र रोग

English-Nepali Medical Glossary – R

Term	Definition	Nepali
ring finger (n)	the third finger from the thumb and next to the little finger	साहिँली औंलो
ringing in the ears (n)	a continuous high pitched noise in the ear, often associated with a history of loud noise exposure	कान बज्नु
ringworm (n)	any of a number of contagious skin diseases caused by several related fungi, characterized by ring-shaped, scaly, itching patches on the skin	दाद
rinse (v)	to wash lightly with water	कुल्ला गर्नु
risk behaviors (n)	activities that may increase the chance of disease or injury	जोखिमयुक्त बानिहरु
root canal (n)	a dental procedure that removes an infected part of a tooth	दाँतको उपचार
root of hair (n)	the portion of the hair that connects to the skin and holds the rest of the hair in place	कपालको जरा
rough (adj)	having a bumpy, uneven surface; not smooth or even	खस्रो
rubdown (n)	an energetic massage of the body	मालीस
rubella (n)	an acute, infectious respiratory and lymphatic system disease; producing a temporary rash; measles	रातो बिबिरा
runny nose (n)	a condition in which excess mucus is present in the nasal cavity, usually caused by an illness, nasal sinus infection, or allergy	रसाएको नाक
rupture (n)	forcible tearing or disruption of tissue; a hernia	फुट्नु

English-Nepali Medical Glossary – S

Term	Definition	Nepali
safe sex (n)	sexual intercourse using contraceptive, usually a condom	सुरक्षित यौन संबंध
safety lock (n)	of, relating to, or containing salt; salty	सुरक्षा ताला
saline (n)	a solution, esp. one that is the same concentration as blood and is used in medicine and surgery	सलाइन
saline abortion (n)	an abortion caused by injecting saline into the womb; used in later stages of pregnancy	सलाइनले गर्भपतन गराउने
saliva (n)	the watery, tasteless liquid mixture released in the mouth	र्याल
salivary glands (n)	special glands in the mouth that secrete saliva and assist in digestion of food	र्याल ग्रन्थी
salivation (n)	the secretion of saliva in the mouth	र्याल निकाल्ने
salpingitis (n)	inflammation of the 1. fallopian or 2. Eustachian tubes	डिम्बबाहिनी नलीको सुजन
salve (n)	a medicinal ointment; something that soothes or heals; balm	मलम
sample (n)	a portion, piece, or segment that is representative of a whole	नमुना
sanatorium (n)	an institution for the treatment of chronic disease	जिर्ण रोगको अस्पताल
sanitary napkins (n)	a disposable pad of absorbent material worn to absorb menstrual flow	सैनिटरी नैपकिन
satisfactory condition (n)	an indication that a patient is doing well and is not in serious danger	संतोषजनक स्थिति
scab (n)	the crust-like skin that covers a healing wound	घाउको पाप्रा

Term	Definition	Nepali
scabies (n)	infestation of the skin by the human itch mite, Sarcaptes; the initial symptom of scabies is the appearance of red, raised bumps that are intensely itchy	लुतो
scald (v)	to burn with or as if with hot liquid or steam	खुइल्याउनु
scale (n)	a dry, thin flake of shedding skin	कत्ला
scalp (n)	the skin covering the top of the human head	टाउकोको छाला
scaly, dry (adj)	covered or partially covered with scales	कत्ले, सुक्खा
scapula (n)	either of two large, flat, triangular bones forming the back part of the shoulder	पाताको हड्डी
scar (n)	a mark left on the skin following the healing of a surface of an injury or wound	खत
Scarlet Fever (n)	an acute contagious disease occurring predominantly among children and characterized by a red skin eruption and high fever	स्कार्लेट ज्वरो
schizophrenia (n)	a mental disorder which causes severe confusion	किजोफ्रेनिया
sciatica (n)	radiating pain from the buttock down the leg	कटिस्नायुशूल
sclera (n)	the white portion of the eye that makes up the outer layer of the eyeball	श्वेतपटल
sclerosis (n)	a thickening or hardening of a body part, as of an artery, esp. from tissue hardening, disease, or overgrowth	कठोरीकरण
scoliosis (n)	abnormal lateral curvature of the spine or back bone	स्कोलियोसिस
scraping (n)	a small piece or bit; fragment	टुक्रा

Term	Definition	Nepali
scratch (v)	1. to make a thin, shallow cut or mark on a surface with a sharp instrument; 2. to rub or scrape the skin to relieve itching	कोतर्नु
screening test (n)	any of various methods use to detect a disease in healthy people	छनोट परीक्षा
scrotum (n)	the external sac of skin enclosing the testes	अण्डाशय
scrub (surgically) (v)	to rub hard in order to clean	सफाई गर्नु (शल्यक्रियाले)
seafood (n)	any food products that come from the water, including shellfish, sea mammals, and fish	सामुद्रीक भोजन
seat belt (n)	a belt used to secure an individual in his or her seat	सिटको पेटी
sebaceous gland (n)	a gland that secretes oil	चिल्लो निकाल्ने ग्रन्थी
secondary care (n)	health care necessary to supplement primary care to meet the enrollee's needs, requiring the knowledge of a physician who is a specialist	कम महत्वपूर्ण रेखदेख
second-hand smoke (n)	environmental tobacco smoke that is inhaled involuntarily or passively by someone who is not smoking; environmental tobacco smoke is generated from the side stream (the burning end) of a cigarette, pipe or cigar or from the exhaled mainstream (the smoke puffed out by smokers) of cigarettes, pipes, and cigars	निष्क्रिय धूम्रपान
secrete (v)	to generate and separate out a substance from cells or bodily fluids; to release a fluid or substance	श्राव उत्पन्न गर्नु

English-Nepali Medical Glossary – S

Term	Definition	Nepali
secretion (n) (m)	1. the act of generating or separating out a substance from cells or bodily fluids; 2. the result of this process	श्राव
sedative (n)	an agent which decreases excitement	शान्त गराउने औषधि
sedentary (adj)	of, or pertaining to a condition of little movement or constant sitting	बसेको
segment (n)	portion of a larger body or structure	खण्ड
seizure (n)	a sudden convulsion and involuntary movement of the body	आक्रमण ?? ~~इस्मठाग~~
selectivity (n)	the degree to which a dose of a drug produces a desired effect	चयनात्मकता
semen (n)	a whitish secretion of the male reproductive organs, the transporting medium for spermatozoa or sperm	वीर्य
seminal vesicles (n)	glandular structures that secrete most of the components of semen	वीर्यथैली
senility (n)	the physical and mental deterioration associated with old age	बुढ्यौली
sensation (n)	a perception associated with stimulation of a sense organ or with a specific bodily condition; the faculty to feel and perceive	अनुभूति
sense (v)	to become aware of; to perceive	चाल पाउनु
sensitive (adj)	capable of perceiving with a sense or the senses	संवेदनशील
sensory (adj)	of, or pertaining to any organ used to feel, sense, smell, hear, see, or detect any sensation	संवेदनात्मक

English-Nepali Medical Glossary – S

Term	Definition	Nepali
septic (adj)	produced by or due to decomposition by microorganisms	दुषित
septicemia (n)	blood poisoning, bacterial infection in the blood	रक्तविषाक्तता
serious condition (n)	a physical or mental condition that could lead to death or considerable damage	गंभीर स्थिति
seroconversion (n)	the development of detectable specific antibodies as a result of a disease or immunization	सेरोकन्भर्जन
serology (n)	the medical science of studying different fluids to detect the presence of antibodies to specific antigens	सीरम विज्ञान
serum (n)	the clear portion of any body fluid	सीरम
sex (n)	1. the condition or character of being male or female; the physiological, functional, and psychological differences that distinguish the male and the female; 2. sexual intercourse	यौन
sexual relations (n)	an encounter characterized by sexual contact	यौन सम्बन्ध
sexually transmitted disease (n)	a contagious disease passed between people during sexual contact	यौन सम्बन्धबाट सर्ने रोग
sharp (adj)	any of various instruments that have a thin edge or a fine point, such as a razor or scalpel	तिखो
shin (n)	having a thin edge or a fine point; suitable for or capable of cutting or piercing; a cutting quality as in pain	धारिलो
shinbone (n)	the tibia; the larger bone between the foot and knee	घुँडामुन्तिरको हड्डी

English-Nepali Medical Glossary – S

Term	Definition	Nepali
shingles (n) (m)	a viral infection causing a line of painful blisters along a nerve path	भैंसे दाद
shiver(v)	to shudder or shake from or as if from cold; to tremble	काम्नु
shock (n) (m)	a generally temporary state of massive bodily trauma, usually characterized by marked loss of blood pressure	झट्का
shock (n) (m)	the sensation and muscular spasm caused by an electric current passing through the body or through a bodily part	आघात, हानी
shock (v)	to give a shock	झट्का लाग्नु
shortness of breath (n)	inability to inhale the necessary amount of air; low energy level due to reduced respiratory rate	सासफेर्न समस्या हुनु
shot (n) (m)	an injection of a drug into a vein, the skin, or muscle	सुई
shot (n) (m)	gun shot	गोली
shoulder (n)	the part of the human body between the neck and upper arm	काँध
shunt (n)	to turn to one side; to divert; to bypass	मार्ग बदल्ने कार्य
siblings (n)	brother or sister; related to one or both parents	भाई बहिनी
side (n)	the left or right half of the trunk of a human	पक्ष
side effect (n)	a secondary effect, esp. an undesirable secondary effect of a drug or therapy	अवांछित प्रभाव
sight (n)	the ability to see	दृष्टि
sigmoid colon (n)	the curving end-section of the large intestine	ठुलो आन्द्राको खण्ड
sigmoidoscope (n)	a slender instrument used to examine the area of the colon closest to the anus	सिग्मोइडोस्कोप

English-Nepali Medical Glossary – S

Term	Definition	Nepali
sign (n) (m)	something that suggests the presence or existence of a fact, condition, or quality, esp. the physical or mental conditions that assist in diagnosing a disease	संकेत
simultaneous (adj)	existing or occurring at the same time	एकैसाथ
sinus (n)	a depression or cavity formed by a bending or curving, esp. in the nose or in the heart; air passage behind the nose and face	शिरानाल
sinusitis (n)	inflammation of the sinus membrane, esp. in the nasal region	पिनास
skeletal system (n)	the entire collection of bone, connective tissue, and cartilage that supports the body and aids in its movement	कंकाल प्रणाली
skilled nursing facility (n)	a health facility that provides continuous skilled nursing care and supportive care to patients whose primary need is for the availability of 24-hour inpatient care	कुशल नर्सिंग सुविधा
skin (n)	the tissue forming the external covering of the body	त्वचा
skin test (n)	any of various tests involving pricking the skin to diagnose a disease, esp. tuberculosis	त्वचा परीक्षण
skull (n)	the bones of the head that make up the brain case and face	खोपडी
sleep disorder (n)	any of various conditions that cause difficulties while sleeping	निन्द्राको बिमारी
sleep inducing (adj)	of, or pertaining to an agent that causes or forces sleep	निन्द्रा लगाउने
sleep walking (n)	the state of walking or movement on one's feet while still apparently sleeping	निन्द्रामा हिंड्ने

English-Nepali Medical Glossary – S

Term	Definition	Nepali
sleeping pills (n)	a sedative, esp. in the form of a pill or capsule, to relieve the inability to sleep	निन्द्रा लगाउने गोली
sling (n)	a looped rope, strap, or chain for supporting, cradling, or hoisting something, esp. a support for a limb when broken or dislocated	काम्रो
slipped disk (n)	the abnormal movement of tissue between vertebrae in the backbone	हड्डी फुस्केको
sliver (n)	a thin piece cut, split, or broken off, esp. a sliver of metal or wood	छेस्को
slurred speech (n)	the act of speaking indistinctly by running sounds together	लर्बरिएको बोली
small intestine (n)	the part of the intestine, extending from the stomach to the large intestine, in which digestion is completed	सानो आन्द्रा
smell (v)	to perceive the scent of something	गन्ध लिनु
smoke (v)	to draw in and exhale the smoke of something, such as tobacco	धुम्रपान गर्नु
smoke detector (n)	a fire safety device in a building or home that makes noise in the presence of smoke	धुवाँ पत्ता लगाउने यन्त्र
smoking cessation (n)	the act of quitting smoking	धूम्रपान रोक्नु
snacks (n)	any prepared food eaten between meals	खाजाहरु
sneeze (v)	to expel air forcibly from the mouth and nose in an explosive, spasmodic involuntary action	हाच्छिउँ गर्नु
sniffles (n)	a condition that prompts someone to sniff repeatedly, as in crying or having a runny nose	सूँ-सूँ गर्नु
snore (v)	to breathe noisily and forcefully through the nose, usually while sleeping	घुर्नु

English-Nepali Medical Glossary – S

Term	Definition	Nepali
soak (v)	to make thoroughly wet or saturated by or as if by placing in liquid	भिजाउनु
soap (n)	a cleansing agent, manufactured in bars, flakes, or liquid form	साबुन
Social Security Administration (n)	the agency of Health and Human Services responsible for the social security system	सामाजिक सुरक्षा प्रशासन
social security number (n)	the number of a particular individual's social security account.	सामाजिक सुरक्षा संख्या
Social Services Agency (n)	the agency responsible for administering state, federal, and county programs for health care, social services, public assistance, job training, and rehabilitation	सामाजिक सेवा एजेंसी
Social Worker (n)	a professional that works within social services	सामाजिक कार्यकर्ता
sodium (n)	a metallic element essential for human life and important in muscle activity, found in table salt and in fast foods in high levels	सोडियम
soft tissue (n)	the tissue including muscle, ligaments, tendons, skin, and fat	नरम तन्तु
sole (n)	the under-surface of the foot	पैताला
solid food (n)	food that does not dissolve readily into liquid form; food that requires chewing	ठोस आहार
somatic (n)	pertaining to the body or body wall	शरीरको
somnolence (n)	sleepiness; unnatural drowsiness	तन्द्रा
sonogram (n)	ultrasonogram; echogram; image obtained by using ultrasound	सोनोग्राम
sonographer (n)	a technologist trained to use ultrasound equipment	सोनोग्राफार

English-Nepali Medical Glossary – S

Term	Definition	Nepali
soporific (n)	causing or inducing sleep; also see *sleep inducing* and *sleeping pills*	निन्द्रा लगाउने
sore (n)	an area painful to touch	पीडादायक
sore throat (n)	any of various inflammations of the tonsils, pharynx, or larynx characterized by pain in swallowing	घाँटी दुख्नु
Spanish (n)	the Romance language of the largest part of Spain and of the countries colonized by Spaniards	स्पेनको
spasm (n)	a sudden, violent, involuntary contraction of a muscle	ऐंठन
spasmodic (adj)	of, or pertaining to an involuntary movement	ऐंठनयुक्त
specialist (n)	a doctor who focuses his or her practice of medicine on one organ or area	विशेषज्ञ
specific (adj)	special, distinctive, or unique, as a quality or attribute	विशिष्ट
specimen (n)	an individual, item, or part taken as representative of an entire set or whole; sample	नमूना
speculum (n)	1. a mirror or polished metal plate used as a reflector; 2. an instrument for widening the opening of a body cavity for medical examination	फट्याउने औजार
spell (n)	1.a short period of time; 2. an access of disease as in fainting spell	अवधि
sperm (n)	spermatozoon; the male contribution to pregnancy	शुक्राणु
spermicide (n)	an agent that is destructive to sperm	शुक्राणुनासक

English-Nepali Medical Glossary – S

Term	Definition	Nepali
sphincter (n) (m)	band of muscles that constrict any passage, as in the stomach or anus	औंठीपेशी
sphygmomanometer (n)	an instrument used to measure blood pressure; also see *blood pressure cuff*	रक्तचाप मापक यन्त्र
spinal anesthesia (n)	anesthetic that is injected into the spinal cord	ढाडको हड्डीमा दिइने एनेस्थीसिया
spinal column (n)	the column of bones enclosing the spinal cord; backbone	मेरुदण्ड
spinal cord (n)	the part of the central nervous system contained within the spinal canal and extending from the brain down the back bone	सुषुम्ना नाडी
spine (n)	the combined nerves, cartilage, and bone that comprise the backbone; the columnar assemblage of connecting vertebrae extending from the head to the pelvis, forming the support axis of the body	मेरुदण्ड
spirometry (n)	a technique of measuring the volume of air entering and leaving the lungs	स्पाइरोमेट्री
spit (n) (m)	saliva, esp. expelled from the mouth	थुक
spit (v) (m)	to eject liquid from the mouth	थुक्नु
spleen (n)	an organ on the left side of the abdomen below the diaphragm that produces white blood cells, filters blood and stores blood cells	फियो
splinter (n)	a sharp, slender piece, as of wood, bone, glass, or metal, split or broken off from the main body	चोइटो
spores (n)	a microorganism such as bacteria that is easily reproduced and can cause the spread of disease	बीजाणू

English-Nepali Medical Glossary – S

Term	Definition	Nepali
spotting (n)	a slight bloody discharge from the vagina	योनीश्राव
sprain (v)	to cause a painful wrenching of the ligaments of a joint	मर्काउनु
sprained (adj)	pertaining to an injury caused by a sprain	मर्केको
spread (v)	to move to other locations within the body	फैलाउनु
sputum (n)	matter ejected through the mouth from the lungs, bronchi, and trachea	खकार
squamous (adj)	scaly or platelike; usually referring to tissues of the skin or the lining of tubes	कत्ले
squeeze (v)	to press together; to compress	निचोर्नु
stab (v)	to pierce or wound with or as if with a pointed object; to plunge a weapon into the body	धस्नु
stable (adj)	of, or pertaining to a physical or mental condition that is not changing	स्थिर
stable condition (n)	the medical condition or state of a patient when a disease or injury no longer threatens the patient's life	स्थिर अवस्था
standard dosing (n)	an established model of administering medication	प्रमाणिक मात्रा दिनु
standards (n)	authoritative statements of (1) minimum levels of acceptable performance or results, (2) excellent levels of performance or results or (3) the range for acceptable performance or results	मापदण्डहरु
stapes (n)	a small bone in the middle ear that assists in hearing	कानको भित्र हुने सानो हड्डी
stay still (v)	to not move; to relax	स्थिर रहनु

English-Nepali Medical Glossary – S

Term	Definition	Nepali
steady state (n)	a condition of not changing	अपरिवर्तित
sterile (adj)	1. incapable of reproducing sexually; infertile; 2. free of bacteria	बाँझो
sterility (n)	1. inability to produce offspring; 2. state of being clean and/or free of bacteria	बाँझोपन
sterilization (n)	1. a surgical procedure that prevents someone from reproducing; 2. complete destruction or elimination of all living micro-organisms	बन्ध्याकरण, सङ्क्रमण मुक्त पार्ने काम
sterilize (v)	1. to make someone sterile; 2. to clean an instrument in such a way that it is free of bacteria	बन्ध्याकरण गर्नु, सङ्क्रमण मुक्त पार्नु
sternum (n)	a long flat bone articulating with the cartilage of and forming the front support for the ribs; breast plate	छातीको हाड
steroid (n)	a specific chemical compound involved in proper body function	स्टेरोइड
stethoscope (n)	an instrument used for listening to sounds produced within the body	स्टेथेस्कोप
stick out your tongue (v)	to make the tongue visible to a physician for examination	जिब्रो बाहिर निकाल्नु
stiff (adj)	difficult to bend or stretch; rigid	कडा
stiffness (n)	the condition of being difficult to bend or stretch	कडापन
stillborn (adj)	dead at birth	जन्मेकै बेलामा मरेको
stimulant (n)	something that temporarily arouses or accelerates activity	उत्तेजक
stimulate (v)	to excite or make active	उत्तेजित पार्नु

English-Nepali Medical Glossary – S

Term	Definition	Nepali
sting (of an insect) (n)	to pierce or wound painfully with or as if with a sharp-pointed structure or organ, such as that of certain insects	टोकाई (किराको)
stitches (n)	1. a series of loops of thread through the skin used to hold a wound closed; 2. sharp, stabbing pains	टाँकाहरु
stomach (n)	the enlarged, saclike portion of the digestive system between the esophagus and small intestine	पेट
stomach ache (n)	pain in the abdomen	पेट दुख्नु
stomach lining (n)	the thick tissue that protects the inside of the stomach	पेटको झिल्ली
stone (n) (m)	mineral matter originating in the kidney, urethra, gallbladder, or bladder	पत्थरी
stool (n)	feces; human waste excreted from the anus	दिसा
stool culture (n)	a test used to detect pathogenic organisms in a sample of feces	दिसा बाट जीबाणु उमार्ने
stool specimen (n)	a sample of feces or bowel movement used to diagnose disease	दिसाको नमुना
strain (v)	to violently stretch or overexert one's muscles	तनक्क पार्नु
strained muscle (n)	a muscle damaged by over use or exercise	क्षति भएको मांशपेशी
strengthening (v)	making stronger	बलियो पार्ने कार्य
strep throat (n)	a specific bacterial infection causing a sore throat	गलाको संक्रामण
stress (n)	forcibly exerted influence; pressure	तनाव
stress test, exercise treadmill test (n)	a method of evaluating the fitness of a patient, esp. the condition of his/her heart	तनाव परीक्षण, व्यायाम ट्रेडमिल परीक्षण

Term	Definition	Nepali
stretch (v)	to flex the muscles of the human body	तन्काउनु
stretcher (n)	a piece of equipment used to transport sick, wounded, or dead people	स्ट्रेचर
stroke (n)	sudden impairment of blood flow to the brain causing paralysis and damage to the brain	आघात
stuffy nose (n)	a blocked nasal passage causing difficulties in breathing	बन्द नाक
stupor (n)	partial or nearly complete unconsciousness	अचेतनता
sty (n)	inflammation of one of the glands in the eyelid	आँखाको ग्रन्थिको सुजन
subcontract (n)	any agreement entered into by a plan for any services necessary to meet the requirements of their original contract	सह-ठेक्का
substance abuse (n)	misuse of substances ranging from nicotine (tobacco) and alcohol to other addictive substances such as barbiturates, narcotics, prescription drugs, and the like	मादक पदार्थको सेवन
suck (v)	to draw air or liquid into the mouth by inhalation or suction; to draw in by or as if by suction	चुस्नु
suction curettage (n)	a type of abortion which removes an unborn fetus by using suction	चूषण गर्भपात
Sudden Infant Death Syndrome (SIDS) (n)	the sudden and unexpected death of a baby with no known illness, typically affecting sleeping infants between the ages of two weeks to six months	सडेन इनफ्यान्ट डेथ सिन्ड्रोम (एस.आइ.डी.एस.)
suffer (v)	to feel or sense pain or discomfort	पिडीत हुनु
suffocate (v)	to impair or prevent respiration; to choke	निसास्सिनु

English-Nepali Medical Glossary – S

Term	Definition	Nepali
suicide (n)	the act or an instance of intentionally killing oneself	आत्महत्या
sunburn (n)	an inflammation or blistering of the skin caused by overexposure to direct sunlight	घामले पोलेको
swallow (v)	to cause something, such as food, to pass through the mouth and throat into the stomach	निल्नु
sweat (n) (m)	perspiration or liquid that is excreted through the pores in the skin	पसीना
sweat (v) (m)	to excrete perspiration or liquid through the pores in the skin	पसीना निकाल्नु
sweets (n)	candy; dessert; any of various foods very high in sugar; also see *carbohydrates*	मिष्ठान्न
swell (v)	to increase in size or volume as a result of internal pressure	सुन्नीनु
swelling (n)	something that has increased in volume due to internal pressure	सुन्नीएको
swollen (adj)	of, or pertaining to something that has increased in volume due to internal pressure	सुन्नीएको
symptom (n)	any subjective evidence of disease or of a patient's condition	लक्षण
symptomatic (adj)	pertaining to, or of the nature of a symptom	लाक्षणिक
syncope (n)	a loss of consciousness caused by a lack of oxygen to the brain, often caused by a heart condition or low blood pressure	बेहोशी
syndrome (n)	a set of symptoms which occur together	सिंड्रोम, लक्षणहरु
syphilis (n)	a chronic infectious disease transmitted by direct contact, usually in sexual intercourse	भिरिंगी

Term	Definition	Nepali
syringe (n)	a medical instrument used to inject fluids into the body or draw them from it	पचका
systemic (adj)	of, or pertaining to the entire body	आंगिक
systole (n)	a single contraction of the heart; the moment blood is ejected from the heart	मुटु खालि हुँदाको अवस्था
systolic (adj)	1. of, or pertaining to a contraction of the heart and the moment blood is ejected from the heart; 2. referring to the higher number in a blood pressure reading	मुटु खालि हुँदाको अवस्थाको

English-Nepali Medical Glossary – T

Term	Definition	Nepali
tablet (n)	a small flat pellet of medication to be taken by mouth	चक्की
take a deep breath (v)	to inhale as much air as possible; to fill the lungs with air	लामो सास लिनु
take off (v)	to remove something, esp. clothing; to undress	फुकाल्नु
tampon (n)	a plug of absorbent material inserted into a bodily cavity or wound to stop a flow of blood or absorb secretions, usually used during menstruation	रगत थाम्ने गद्दा
tapeworm (n)	any of various ribbon-like, often very long, flatworms that are parasitic and live in the intestines	फित्तेजुका
taste (n)	the sense that distinguishes the flavor of a substance	स्वाद
taste (v)	to distinguish the flavor of a substance	चाख्नु
tea spoon (n)	the common small spoon used esp. with tea, coffee, and desserts; a measurement equal to approximately 5 milliliters, (or 5 cc)	चियाचम्चा
tear (n) (m)	to pull apart or into pieces; to make an opening by ripping; to divide, disunite	आँशु
tear (v) (m)	to secrete liquid from around the eye	आँशु निकाल्नु
tear (v) (m)	a drop of liquid secreted from around the eye	च्यात्नु
tear duct (n)	a canal or channel from the lachrymal gland that secretes a salty liquid commonly called tears	अश्रुनली
technician (n)	an expert in a technique, procedure, or complex task	प्राविधिक
teenager (n)	a person between the ages of 13 and 19; an adolescent	किशोर

English-Nepali Medical Glossary – T

Term	Definition	Nepali
teething (v)	the inflammation when new teeth develop in a baby	दाँत निस्कनु
Telecommunication Device for the Deaf (TDD) (n)	a special type of phone used to communicate with the deaf and hearing impaired	टेलीकम्युनिकेसन डीभाइस फर द डेफ (टि.डी.डी.)
telephone number (n)	a number assigned to a telephone line for a specific location that is used to call that location	टेलिफोन नम्बर
temperature (n)	the degree of hotness or coldness of a body or environment	तापक्रम
temple (n) (m)	the flat region on either side of the forehead	कन्चट
temporary lodging (n)	housing or shelter intended to be used for a limited time	अस्थाई बसोबास
tender (adj)	easily bruised; sensitive; painful or sore	नरम
tendon (n)	a band of tough, inelastic fibrous tissue that connects a muscle with its bony attachment	सन्धिबन्धन
tendonitis (n)	inflammation of tendons and of tendon-muscle attachments	सन्धिबन्धनको सुजन
tennis elbow, golfer's elbow (n)	tendinitis; inflammation of tendons and of tendon-muscle attachments, usually from overuse	सन्धिबन्धनको सुजन
tense (adj)	tightly stretched, strained, esp. tense muscles; in a state of mental or nervous tension or stress	तनावपूर्ण
tension (n)	the condition of being stretched or strained, emotional strain or stress	तनाव
terminal (adj)	1. final; ending; the most distant; 2. severity of a medical condition leading to the end of a patient's life	अन्तिम

English-Nepali Medical Glossary – T

Term	Definition	Nepali
terminally ill (adj)	severity of a patient's medical condition leading to the end of a patient's life	अन्तिम अवस्थाको बिरामी
test (n)	a means of examination, trial, or proof, esp. a medical procedure used to diagnosis a disease	परिक्षण
test of pulmonary function (n)	any of various medical examinations to assess the function of the lungs and assist in diagnosis of diseases of the lungs; also see *pulmonary function tests (PFT)*	फोक्सोको कार्य परिक्षण
test strip (n)	a piece of paper used to determine the acidity of a liquid, or the sugar content of blood	परीक्षण पट्टी
test tube (n)	a clear glass tube usually open at one end and rounded at the closed end, used in laboratory experiments	परीक्षण नली
test tube baby (n)	a baby that has been conceived outside the womb through fertilization of an egg removed from the mother	टेस्ट ट्यूब बेबी
testicle (n)	a testis	अण्डकोष
testicular/prostate problems (n)	medical problems with the testes or prostate gland	अण्डकोष/प्रोस्ट्रेटका समस्याहरु
testis (n)	the male reproductive gland, normally paired in an external scrotum or sac of skin	अण्डकोष
tetanus (n)	an acute, often fatal infectious disease which generally enters the body through wounds	धनुष्टंकार
therapeutic counseling (n)	individual or group counseling to assist with social, psychological, or medical problems	चिकित्सकीय परामर्श
therapeutics (n)	the art of healing, having healing or curative powers	चिकित्सा विज्ञान

English-Nepali Medical Glossary – T

Term	Definition	Nepali
therapy (n)	treatment of disease	उपचार
thermometer (n)	an instrument for measuring temperature	तापक्रम मापक यन्त्र
thigh (n)	the portion of the human leg between the hip and the knee; femur	तिघ्रा
thighbone (n)	the femur; the large bone between the knee and hip	तिघ्राको हड्डी
thoracic (adj)	pertaining to or affecting the chest	छातिको
thorax (n)	the chest and the organs and tissue within it, including the heart, lungs, esophagus, and ribs	छाती
throat (n)	the portion of the digestive tract that lies between the rear of the mouth and the esophagus	गला
throat drops, lozenges (n)	medication administered directly into the throat in drop form or as a candy, used to decrease the irritation of a sore throat	घाँटीदुखेको औषधि
throb (v)	to vibrate, pulsate, or sound rapidly or violently with steady rhythm; to pound	बलक बलक गर्नु
throbbing (adj)	of, or pertaining to something that throbs, esp. in reference to a headache or injury	बल्किने खालको
thrombophlebitis (n)	inflammation of a vein caused by a blood clot	शिराको सुजन
thrombosis (n)	the formation, presence, or development of a blood clot in a blood vessel	रक्तनलीमा रगत जम्नु
thrombus (n)	a blood clot blocking a blood vessel or formed in a heart cavity	रक्तनलीमा जमेको रगत
thrush (n)	a yeast infection sometimes causing white spots in the mouth	मुखमा हुने ढुसीको सङ्क्रमण
thumb (n)	the short first digit of the human hand, opposable to each of the other four digits	बुढीऔंला

English-Nepali Medical Glossary – T

Term	Definition	Nepali
thyroid (n)	a two-lobed gland that produces hormones, located in front of and on either side of the throat in humans	थाईरोइड
thyroid problems (n)	problems related to the thyroid	थाईरोइडका समस्याहरु
thyroid stimulating hormone (n)	thyrotropin; a hormone that stimulates or promotes activity of the thyroid gland and regulates body weight; an elevated thyroid stimulating hormone indicates a low thyroid level	थाईरोइड स्टिमुलेटिंग हर्मोन
thyroid stimulating hormone assay (n)	a test to determine the level of thyroid stimulating hormone in the body	थाईरोइड स्टिमुलेटिंग हर्मोनको परिक्षण
thyroid test (n)	a procedure used to determine the level of hormones released by the thyroid and to assist in diagnosis	थाईरोइड परिक्षण
tibia (n)	the larger of two bones between the knee and ankle	नलीहाड
tick (insect) (n)	any of numerous bloodsucking parasites that transmit infectious diseases	किर्ना
tie the tubes (v)	a surgical procedure that renders a female infertile or unable to become pregnant	महिलाको बन्ध्याकरण
tight (adj)	cramped; constrained; constricted; snug, often uncomfortably so	कस्सिएको
tightness (n)	the condition of being tight	कस्सिएको अवस्था
tinea, ringworm (n)	any of various fungous skin diseases	दाद
tingling (adj)	of, or pertaining to a prickling, stinging sensation, as from cold, a sharp slap, or excitement	झमझामाउने

English-Nepali Medical Glossary – T

Term	Definition	Nepali
tiredness (n)	the condition of being worn-out or fatigued	थकान
tissue (n)	a collection of cells that share a similar function, the soft parts of the body	तन्तु
toddler (n)	a young child between the ages of about one and three years learning to walk	शिशु
toe (n)	one of the digits of the foot	खुट्टाको औंला
toenail (n)	the hard covering on a toe	खुट्टाको औंलाको नङ
tolerance (n)	the ability to endure unusually large doses of a drug or toxin	सहनशिलता
tongue (n)	the fleshy muscular organ, attached to the floor of the mouth, that is the principle organ of taste, an important organ of speech, and that aids chewing and swallowing	जिब्रो
tonometry (n)	the diagnostic procedure that uses an instrument to measure the pressure within the eyeball	टोनोमेट्री
tonsillectomy (n)	surgical removal of the tonsils	टन्सिल हटाउनु
tonsillitis (n)	inflammation of the tonsils	टन्सिलको सुजन
tonsil (n)	a mass of tissue, esp. either of two such masses, embedded in the walls between the mouth and pharynx	टन्सिल
tooth (n)	one of a set of hard, bone-like structures rooted in sockets in the jaws	दाँत
tooth brush (n)	a brush used for cleaning teeth	दाँत माझ्ने ब्रस
tooth decay (n)	the destruction or decomposition of a tooth, usually caused by disease	दाँत सड्नु

English-Nepali Medical Glossary – T

Term	Definition	Nepali
tooth socket (n)	a hollow cavity in which the roots of a tooth are held in place	दाँत अडिने प्वाल
toothache (n)	an aching pain in or near a tooth	दाँत दुख्नु
toothpaste (n)	a paste for cleaning teeth	दन्तमन्जन
topic (n)	a subject or theme of a discussion or conversation	शिर्षक
topical (adj)	pertaining to a particular surface area; of, or applied to an isolated part of the body; something applied to the skin	सतहमा लगाइने
torn (adj)	of, or pertaining to something that has been pulled apart or into pieces, divided, esp. a ligament	च्यातिएको
torsion (n)	a type of mechanical stress where an object is twisted and contorted	बटारिएको
torso (n)	the trunk of the human body	धड
total knee	a surgical procedure that removes a section of the bone around the knee and replaces it with an artificial joint	सबै घुँडा
touch (v)	to feel; to come in contact with something by using a hand or finger	छुनु
tourniquet (n)	a device used to temporarily stop the flow of blood through a large artery in a limb	बन्धन
towel (n)	a piece of cloth used for drying or cleaning	तौलिया
toxemia (n)	condition resulting from the spread of bacterial products in the bloodstream; high blood pressure and seizures caused by pregnancy	रक्त विषाक्तता
toxic (adj)	pertaining to the nature of poison; harmful, destructive, or deadly	बिषालु

English-Nepali Medical Glossary – T

Term	Definition	Nepali
toxicity (n)	quality of being poisonous	विषाक्तता
toxin (n)	a poison	बिष
trachea (n)	a thin-walled tube of cartilage and membrane tissue descending from the larynx to the bronchi and carrying air to the lungs	श्वासनली
tracheitis (n)	inflammation of the trachea	श्वासनलीको सुजन
tracheotomy (n)	the act or procedure of cutting into the trachea through the neck to provide an air passage	श्वासनली काटेर हटाउनु
traction (n)	the act of drawing or pulling	तान्नु
traditional healer (n)	competent to provide health care by using vegetable, animal and mineral substances and certain other methods based on the social, cultural and religious background as well as on the knowledge, attitudes and beliefs that are prevalent in the community regarding physical, mental and social well-being and the causation of disease and disability (The Promotion and Development of Traditional Medicine - TRS 622, WHO, Geneva, 1978)	धामीझाँक्री
trainee (n)	student; resident; a person learning a specific field, technique, or skill	ताहिम लिनेवाल प्रशिक्षार्थी
tranquilize (v)	to calm or reduce mental activity, usually by administering a medication	शान्त पार्नु
tranquilizer (n)	a drug with a calming, soothing effect	शान्त पार्ने औषधि
transdermal (adj)	entering through the skin	छालाबाट छिरेको

English-Nepali Medical Glossary – T

Term	Definition	Nepali
transfusion (n)	introduction of whole blood directly into the blood stream	प्रत्यारोपण
translator (n)	a person who translates written texts	अनुवादक
transplant procedure (n)	an operation in which tissue or an organ is transplanted from one person (the donor) to another (the recipient)	प्रत्यारोप प्रक्रिया
transplantation (n)	the transfer of tissue or an organ from one body, or body part, to another	प्रत्यारोपण
transportation/escort	assistance for clients who require personal care or support while being transported	परिवहन/रक्षा
transportation/regular (n)	assist client to transit to a designated place	परिवहन/नियमित
transverse colon (n)	the middle section of the large intestine	ठुलो आन्द्राको बिचको भाग
trauma (n)	a wound, esp. one produced by sudden physical injury	घाऊ *मानसिक आघात*
traumatic (adj)	relating to or resulting from trauma	घाऊको
treatment (n)	the use or application of remedies with the goal of effecting a cure; therapy	उपचार
tremor (n)	an involuntary trembling or quivering	कम्पन
triggers (n)	allergens such as pollen, dust, or animal dander that cause an asthma episode (attack)	प्रवर्तकहरु
tubal ligation (n)	female sterilization; surgical procedure that prevents a woman from reproducing	महिलाको परिवार नियोजन

English-Nepali Medical Glossary – T

Term	Definition	Nepali
tube (n)	a hollow cylinder, esp. one that conveys a fluid or functions as a passage; any of various tubes or tube-like structures in the human body including the fallopian tubes, the Eustachian tubes, the urethra, and ureter	नली
tuberculine test (n)	any of various tests used to determine past or present infection with a bacteria called tubercle bacillus	क्षयरोगको परिक्षण
tuberculosis (n)	a contagious disease that damages bone, the lungs, and other parts of the body	क्षयरोग
tuberculostatic (adj)	inhibiting the growth of tuberculosis	क्षयरोगको किटाणुनासक
tumor (n)	an abnormal tissue growth	ट्युमर
tunnel vision (n)	a reduced field of vision in which vision is limited to the center; extreme narrow view	सुरुंग दृष्टि
turn over (v)	to move or rotate the entire body in one direction to reveal the back or front side	पल्टनु
tweezers (n)	a small, usually metal, tool used for handling small objects	चिम्टी
twins (n)	two offspring produced in the same pregnancy	जुम्ल्याहा
twitch (n)	a sudden small involuntary movement; jerk	बटारिनु
tympanic membrane (n)	ear drum; a thin membrane that divides the outer ear from the middle ear	मध्यकानको झिल्ली
typhoid fever (n)	an acute, highly infectious disease transmitted by contaminated food or water and characterized by red rashes, high fever, and intestinal bleeding	टाइफाइड

English-Nepali Medical Glossary – U

Term	Definition	Nepali
ulcer (n)	a local defect of the surface of an organ or tissue; an inflammatory cut on the skin or internal surface of the body, often refers to a painful defect in the stomach lining	अल्सर, घाऊ
ulceration (n)	formation or development of an ulcer	घाऊ हुनु
ulna (n)	the bone extending from the elbow to the wrist on the side opposite the thumb	कुहिनो
ultrasound (n)	high frequency sound used in diagnostic imaging of internal organs	अल्ट्रासाउण्ड
Ultraviolet (UV) Protection (n)	protection from the UV radiation of the sun	पराबैजनी (यू.भी.) सुरक्षा
ultraviolet treatment (n)	therapy used to treat psoriasis, a disease causing lesions on the skin, by using ultraviolet radiation	पराबैजनी उपचार
umbilical cord (n)	the flexible, cord-like structure connecting the unborn baby to the mother at the navel; it supplies blood to the baby and removes the baby's waste	नाल
unconscious (adj)	without conscious awareness, asleep and unable to respond to sensory stimuli	बेहोस
underarm (n)	armpit	काखी
undernourished (adj)	the condition of being provided insufficient quantity and quality of food to sustain proper health and growth	कुपोषित
uniform (n)	marked by lack of variation	समान
unilateral (adj)	affecting only one side, esp. one half of the body	एकातर्फी

English-Nepali Medical Glossary – U

Term	Definition	Nepali
unsafe (adj)	harmful or dangerous	असुरक्षित
unwanted (adj)	not wanted, required, or needed	अनावश्यक
upper (adj)	higher in place, position, or rank	माथिल्लो
upper arm (n)	the section of the arm between the shoulder and elbow	पाखुरा
upper respiratory infection (n)	any of various infections of the bronchi, nasal passages, throat, or sinus passages	श्वासप्रश्वास प्रणालीको माथिल्लो भागको सङ्क्रमण
upset stomach (n)	a condition where the stomach is disturbed, not functioning normally, and agitated	पेटको खराबी
ureter (n)	the tube that carries fluid from the kidney to the bladder	मूत्रनली
urethra (n)	the canal through which urine is discharged from the bladder	मुत्रमार्ग
urethroscope (n)	a slender instrument used to visually examine the interior of the urethra	मुत्रमार्गको अवलोकन
urgency (n)	the sudden compelling urge or need to take action, esp. to urinate	आवश्यकता
urgent care (n)	services required to prevent serious deterioration of health following the onset of an unforeseen condition or injury (i.e., sore throats, fever, lacerations, and broken bones)	अत्यावश्यक रेखदेख
uric acid (n)	a product of metabolism found in blood and urine; also see *gout*	यूरिक एसिड
urinalysis (n)	the chemical analysis or examination of urine	मुत्र परीक्षण
urinary (adj)	pertaining to the urine; containing or secreting urine	मुत्र सम्बन्धि
urinary system (n)	the system of organs, tissues, and functions that are involved in urination or the excretion of urine	मुत्र प्रणाली

English-Nepali Medical Glossary – U

Term	Definition	Nepali
urinary tract infection (n)	an infection of the urinary tract with microorganisms	मुत्र मार्गको सङ्क्रमण
urinate (v)	to excrete urine; to discharge water and waste from the bladder	मुत्र त्याग गर्नु
urination (n)	the act of discharging water and waste from the bladder	मुत्र त्याग
urine (n)	the fluid and dissolved substances secreted by the kidneys, stored in the bladder, and excreted from the body through the urethra	मुत्र
urogenital (adj)	pertaining to the urinary and genital apparatus	मुत्र-जनेन्द्रीयको
urologist (n)	the physician who specializes in the physiology and pathology of the genitourinary tract	मुत्र-जनेन्द्रीय विशेषज्ञ
uterine lining (n)	the tissue that lines the inside of the uterus which is lost during menstruation	पाठेघरको झिल्ली
uterus (n)	hollow muscular female organ that holds a developing fetus	पाठेघर
utilization	the rate patterns of service usage or types of service occurring within a specified time. Utilization is generally expressed in rates per unit of population-at-risk for a given period; e.g., the number of admissions to a hospital per 1,000 persons enrolled in an HMO per year	उपयोग
uvula (n)	the small, fleshy mass of tissue suspended from the roof of the mouth above the back of the tongue	किलकिले

English-Nepali Medical Glossary – V

Term	Definition	Nepali
vaccinate (v)	to administer a vaccine in order to prevent a future disease from developing	खोपाउनु
vaccination (n)	introduction of vaccine into the body for the purpose of inducing immunity	खोप कार्य
vaccine (n)	a suspension of a killed microorganism or other substance, injected into the body as prevention against a disease	खोप
Vaccines for Children (VFC) (n)	a government program that offers vaccines at no cost for eligible children through VFC-enrolled doctors	भ्याक्सिन्स फर चिल्ड्रेन (भी.एफ.सी.)
vagina (n)	the passage leading from the uterus to the external female genitalia	योनीमार्ग
vaginal (adj)	pertaining to the vagina	योनीमार्गको
vaginal bleeding (n)	bleeding through the vagina during menstruation, pregnancy, miscarriage, abortion, or tumor	योनीमार्गको रक्तश्राव
vaginal problems (n)	medical problems with a vagina	योनीमार्गको समस्याहरु
vaginal yeast infection (n)	a fungus infection of the vagina that causes irritation	योनीमार्गको ढुसी संक्रमण
vaginitis (n)	inflammation of the vagina	योनीमार्गको सुजन
valve (n) (m)	a membranous structure in a hollow organ or a passage, as in an artery or a vein, that retards or prevents the return flow of a bodily fluid	भल्भ, द्वार
varicose vein (n)	an abnormal swelling of a vein of the leg	शिराशोथ
vascular (adj)	of, pertaining to, characterized by, or containing vessels for the transmission or circulation of fluids, esp. blood	रक्तनली युक्त

English-Nepali Medical Glossary – V

Term	Definition	Nepali
vasculitis (n)	inflammation of a vessel	रक्तनलीको सुजन
vasectomy, male sterilization (n)	surgical procedure that makes a male infertile	भ्यासेक्टोमी, पुरुषहरुको बन्ध्याकरण
vegetative state (n)	coma; a state of involuntary or unconscious functioning, esp. after severe head trauma or brain disease, in which an individual is incapable of voluntary or purposeful acts, and is thought to be unable to think or feel	प्रगाढ बेहोशी
vein (n)	a vessel that transports blood toward the heart	शिरा
vena cava (n)	the large vein in the body that brings blood from the body to the heart	भेनाकाभा
venereal (adj)	pertaining or related to, or transmitted by sexual contact	मैथुन सम्बन्धि
venereal disease (n)	a disease that is transmitted by sexual contact; sexually transmitted disease	यौनरोग
venous (adj)	of, or pertaining to the veins	शिराको
ventilator (n)	breathing machine; an instrument that assists someone's respiration, ensuring that an adequate amount of oxygen reaches the lungs	भेन्टिलेटर
ventricle (n)	either of two muscular chambers of the heart that are responsible for forcing blood away from the heart	मुटुको तल्लो भाग
vertebra (n)	any of the bone segments forming the spinal column or back bone	मेरुदण्डको हाड
vertigo (n)	the sensation of dizziness and the feeling that oneself or one's environment is whirling about	रिंगटा लाग्ने

Term	Definition	Nepali
viral (adj)	pertaining to the nature of virus or symptoms of a virus, esp. in characterizing an infection	बिषाणुजन्य
viral hepatitis (n)	liver infection caused by a virus	बिषाणुजन्य कलेजोको सुजन
viral illness (n)	any of various diseases caused by organisms smaller than can be seen with a microscope	बिषाणुजन्य बिमारी
virus (n)	any of various disease-causing organisms, smaller than can be seen with a microscope, that can enter and reproduce in a cell	बिषाणु
vision (n)	the act or faculty of seeing; sight	दृष्टि
visiting nurse (n)	a nurse that provides health care in the home or outside of a hospital or clinic	भिजिटिङ नर्स
visual fields examination (n)	a procedure used to determine a patient's range of sight or vision, to see if all parts of the eye are seeing properly	भिजुअल फिल्ड्स एक्जामिनेसन
vital capacity (n)	the volume of gas that can be expelled from the lungs after a deep breath	फोक्सोको क्षमता
vitamin (n)	any of various relatively complex substances occurring naturally in plant and animal tissue and essential in small amounts for human metabolism and function	भिटामीन
vitamin supplements (n)	oral medication used to supply the body with essential vitamins that might be at low levels in the body	भिटामीनयुक्त खुराक
vitreous humor (n)	the clear fluid inside the eyeball	भीट्रीएस ह्युमर

English-Nepali Medical Glossary – V

Term	Definition	Nepali
vocal cord (n)	the lower of two pairs of bands or folds in the larynx that vibrate when pulled together and when air is passed up from the lungs, producing sounds and voice	ध्वनीयन्त्र
voice box (n)	the larynx and vocal cords, organs that enable speech	ध्वनीयन्त्र
vomit (n)	matter ejected from the stomach through the mouth	बान्ता
vomit (v)	to eject part or all of the contents of the stomach through the mouth, usually in a series of involuntary muscle contractions	बान्ता गर्नु
vulva (n)	the external female genitalia	योनि
vulvovaginitis (n)	inflammation of the vulva and vagina; vaginitis	योनि र योनिमार्गको सुजन

English-Nepali Medical Glossary – W

Term	Definition	Nepali
waist (n)	the part of the human trunk between the bottom of the rib cage and the pelvis	कमर
waiting room (n)	a place where people can sit and rest while waiting, as in a doctor's office	प्रतिक्षा कक्ष
walker (n)	a frame device used to support a person while walking	वाकर, हिड्न साहयता गर्ने
warm-up (v)	a low-intensity aerobic exercise that involves stretching for 5-10 minutes to prevent muscle and skeletal injuries	हल्का कसरत गर्नु
wart (n)	a small, circular, hard growth on the hands or feet caused by a virus	मुसा
watery eyes (n)	a condition where the lens of the eye is covered with excess fluid secreted from the lachrymal gland, usually caused by an allergic reaction or irritation	रसिलो आँखा
weak (adj)	lacking physical strength, energy, or vigor; likely to fail under pressure, stress, or strain	कमजोर
weak spot (n)	a location or area that has the quality or is in a state of weakness	कमजोर विन्दु
weakness (n)	the condition of being weak	कमजोरी
wean (v)	to withhold mother's milk from the young and substitute other food; to slowly reduce a treatment	दुध छुटाउनु
weight (over, under, gain, lose) (n)	a measurement of heaviness or mass of a person	तौल (बढ्नु, घट्नु, तल, माथि)
weight management (n)	a program based on eating a balanced diet, getting regular exercise, and learning to feel good about your body	तौल ब्यबस्थापन

English-Nepali Medical Glossary – W

Term	Definition	Nepali
welfare (n)	the provision of economic or social benefits to a certain group of people, esp. aid furnished by the government or by private agencies to the needy or disabled	कल्याण
well care visit schedule (n)	a schedule of well-care visits for children as recommended by the American Academy of Pediatrics (AAP)	वेल केयर भिजिट सेड्युल
wet the bed (v)	to urinate unknowingly or involuntarily while sleeping	ओछ्यान भिजाउनु
wheals (n)	an acute swelling or thickening of the skin	एक्कासी सुनिनु
wheelchair (n)	a chair mounted on large wheels used to assist a person who is sick, disabled, or incapable of walking	व्हीलचेयर
wheeze (v)	to breathe with difficulty, producing a hoarse whistling sound	स्वाँ स्वाँ गर्नु
white blood cells (n)	cells found in the blood that are responsible for fighting infection and disease; leukocytes	श्वेत रक्तकोष
whooping cough (n)	an infectious disease involving the respiratory passages and characterized by spasms of coughing with deep, noisy inspiration; pertussis	लहरेखोकी
WIC (Special Supplemental Nutrition Program for Women, Infants & Children) (n)	health care referrals, and nutrition education to pregnant women, new mothers, and their infants	डब्लु.आइ.सी.(स्पेसल सप्लिमेन्टल न्युट्रीसन प्रोग्राम फर विमेन, इन्फेन्ट्स एण्ड चिल्ड्रेन)
windpipe (n)	airway; trachea; the passage through which air reaches the lungs	श्वासनली

Term	Definition	Nepali
wisdom tooth (n)	one of four molars, the last teeth on each side of both jaws, usually appearing later than other teeth	बुद्धिबंगारो
withdrawal (n)	1. the act or process of removing or taking away; 2. symptoms experienced when an addictive substance is stopped	हात झिक्ने काम
womb (n)	the uterus; a hollow muscular female organ that holds a developing fetus	पाठेघर
work related injury (n)	an injury caused by or occurring at work	काम गर्दा लागेको चोट
work release (n)	documentation provided by a doctor that states the patient is capable of performing specific work	काम स्वतन्त्रता
World Health Organization (WHO) (n)	a United Nations agency that coordinates international health activities and helps governments improve health services	विश्व स्वास्थ्य संगठन (डब्ल्यू.एच.ओ.)
worry (v)	to feel uneasy about; to be troubled	चिन्ता
wound (n)	an injury, esp. one in which the skin is torn, pierced, cut, or otherwise broken	चोट, घाऊ
wrist (n)	the junction between the hand and forearm	नारी

English-Nepali Medical Glossary – XYZ

Term	Definition	Nepali
x-ray (n) (m)	a photograph created by x-ray imaging of bone and internal organs	एक्स-रे
x-ray (v) (m)	to photograph with x-rays used in diagnostic imaging of bone and internal organs	एक्स-रे गर्नु
yawn (n)	a large inhalation of air while holding the mouth wide open, esp. when tired or needing sleep	मुख बाउनु
yeast (n)	any of various single-cell fungi that reproduce by budding and are capable of fermenting sugars	ढुसी
yeast infection (n)	infection caused by yeast, often vaginal	ढुसीको सङ्क्रमण
yellow fever (n)	an acute infectious disease transmitted by mosquitos, causing vomiting and yellow coloring of the skin	पितज्वरो
zinc (n)	a mineral essential for proper body function	जिंक

The Medical Team

English	Nepali
Advanced Registered Nurse Practitioner (ANRP)	एडभान्स्ड-रजिस्टर्ड नर्स प्राक्टिसनर
Anesthetist	बेहोसीको औषधि दिने व्यक्ति
Attending Physician	कार्यवाहक चिकित्सक
Certified Nurse Midwife	सर्टिफाइड नर्स मिडवाइफ
Counselor	परामर्शदाता
Doctor	चिकित्सक
Family Doctor	चिकित्सक
Licensed Practical Nurse (LPN)	लाइसन्स प्राप्त नर्स
Nutritionist	पोषणविद्
Pediatrician	बाल चिकित्सक
Pharmacist	औषधि विक्रेता
Physical Therapist	शारीरिक चिकित्सक
Psychiatrist	मनोचिकित्सक
Psychologist	मनोवैज्ञानिक
Receptionist	रिसेप्शनिस्ट
Registered Nurse (RN)	पंजीकृत नर्स
Social Worker	सामाजिक कार्यकर्ता
Surgeon	शल्यचिकित्सक
Visiting Nurse	भिजिटिङ नर्स

Medical Specialists

English	Nepali
Cardiologist	मुटुरोग विज्ञ, मुटुरोग बिषेशज्ञ
Dermatologist	छालाको चिकित्सक
Endocrinologist	एंडोक्राइनोलॉजिस्ट, अन्त:श्राव रोग विशेषज्ञ
Gastroenterologist	पेटरोग विशेषज्ञ
Gynecologist	स्त्रीरोग विशेषज्ञ
Obstetric Nurse	प्रसूति नर्स
Obstetrician	प्रसूति विज्ञ
Ophthalmologist	नेत्र विशेषज्ञ
Optometrist	ओप्टोमेट्रीस्ट
Orthodontist	दन्त विशेषज्ञ
Orthopedist	हाडजोर्नी विशेषज्ञ
Pathologist	रोगविज्ञ
Pulmonologist	फोक्सोको विशेषज्ञ
Radiologist	रेडियोलोजीस्ट

Medical Procedures and Exams

English	Nepali
Biopsy	बायोप्सी
Blood Test	रक्त परिक्षण
Bone Scan	हड्डीको तस्विर लिने काम
Catheterization	शरीरभित्र नली घुसार्ने काम
Colonoscopy	ठुलो आन्द्राको अवलोकन
Computerized Axial Tomography (CAT Scan)	क्याट स्क्यान, सी.टि. स्क्यान
Electrocardiogram	मुटुको बिद्युतिय गतिविधिको रेखा-चित्र
Electroencephalography	दिमागको बिद्युतिय गतिविधिको रेखा-चित्र लिने कार्य
Injection	सूई
Lumbar Puncture, Spinal Tap	ढाडमा सियो घुसार्ने काम
Magnetic Resonance Imaging	म्याग्नेटिक रिजोनेन्स इमेजिंग
Needle Aspiration Biopsy	निडल एस्पाईरेसन बायोप्सी
Operation	शल्यक्रिया
Stress Test, Exercise Treadmill Test	तनाव परीक्षण, व्यायाम ट्रेडमिल परीक्षण
Surgery	शल्यचिकित्सा
Ultrasound	अल्ट्रासाउण्ड
X-Ray	एक्स-रे गर्नु

Types of Pain

English	Nepali
Ache	दुख्नु
Burning Pain	पोलाईले गर्दा दुख्नु
Constant Pain	लगातारको पिडा
Cramp	ऐंठन
Dull Pain	हल्का पिडा
On and Off Pain	यदाकदा हुने पिडा
Pain	पिडा
Radiating Pain	फैलेको पिडा
Sharp Pain	कडा पिडा
Shooting Pain	एक्कासी भएको पिडा
Throbbing Pain	बल्किएको पिडा

Medical Equipment

English	Nepali
Bandage	पट्टि
Bedpan	कोपरा
Blood Pressure Cuff	रक्तचाप नाप्ने यन्त्र
Brace	काँटा लगाएर अड्याउनु
Cast (Plaster)	लगाइएको प्लास्टर
Catheter	शरीरभित्र घुसाइने नली
Forceps	चिम्टा
Gauze	पट्टि
Monitor	मनिटर
Needle, Syringe	सूई, सियो
Otoscope	ओटोस्कोप
Rhinoscope	राइनोस्कोप
Speculum	फट्याउने औजार
Stethoscope	स्टेथेस्कोप
Ventilator	भेन्टिलेटर

Made in the USA
Columbia, SC
14 July 2018